Infection Control

in the former

Wet Finger Environment

by
Robert R. Runnells, D.D.S.
Clinical Assistant Professor
University of Utah School of Medicine
Department of Pathology

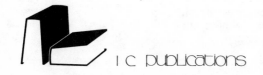

IC PUBLICATIONS

First Edition
November 1987

Acknowledgements

This book was originally intended as a second edition of *INFECTION CONTROL IN THE WET FINGER ENVIRONMENT,* the first work published by the author in 1984; however, as revisions began, it became apparent that the field of infection control had moved so rapidly in the past three years that more than a second edition was needed. Perhaps the most dramatic change in dental infection control was the evolution from "wet finger" to "gloved hands" dentistry. The new title incorporating the words "former wet finger environment" is intended to emphasize the obvious change of bare-handed dentistry to gloved-handed dentistry *and* the many other infection control procedures implemented in the dental environment.

Many of the reviewing editors of the original *"WET FINGER"* book have continued to work closely with the author as the new text has evolved. While not directly editing this new text, these past reviewers should be recognized for their many constructive comments and contributions through the past three years.

While many persons have contributed indirectly to the subject matter, the author wishes to particularly thank the following persons for their contributions above and beyond the call of duty:

L.W. Miltenberger, Jr., D.D.S., *University of Utah*
James A. Cottone, D.M.D., M.S., *University of Texas Health Science Center, Dental School, San Antonio*
James J. Crawford, Ph.D., *University of North Carolina*
Cris Edwards, C.D.A., *Littleton, Colorado*
Frank B. Engley, Jr., Ph.D., *University of Missouri*
Bruce A. Matis, D.D.S., M.S.D., *School of Aerospace Medicine, Brooks AFB, Texas*
Chris H. Miller, Ph.D., *Indiana University School of Medicine*
John A. Molinari, Ph.D., *University of Detroit School of Dentistry*
G. Lynn Powell, D.D.S., *University of Utah*
Milton E. Schaefer, D.D.S., M.L.A., *University of So. California School of Dentistry*
Robert J. Whitacre, M.S., D.D.S., *Seattle, Washington*

Most of all, I thank my wife, Marian, who has been understanding, supportive, and encouraging.

R.R.R.

The purpose of this workbook is to make dental infection control more understandable and, thereby, make a higher level of patient care more attainable. Following are the primary objectives of the work:

1. To emphasize the need for a PRACTICAL program of control to protect patients and staff from infection in the dental office.

2. To provide sufficient credible scientific data to underscore the very real need for an efficacious infection control program.

3. To outline a logical step-by-step program of control which can be utilized in a busy office without the compromising of the multitude of other demands inherent in the practice of dentistry.

4. To motivate office staff to become conscientiously involved in a continuously evolving program.

5. To provide a learning aid useful to the widest audience, from the experienced dentist to the newly hired, inexperienced assistant, with each reader being treated as a mature individual.

The quick reference charts are intended to be placed on the wall to serve as constant reminders of points or procedures which might otherwise be overlooked or forgotten.

No pretense is made to a thorough review of parts of the subject, particularly of the basic sciences. The use of more exhaustive and specific textbooks on these subjects is suggested.

Quoted sources and suggested readings have been compiled into a sequential list at the end of each chapter to correspond with consecutively numbered references within the text.

It is my sincere hope that the reader will find the information comprehensible and useful.

R.R.R.

Table of Contents

CHAPTER 1

The "I've Never Had A Problem" Problem

ABSTRACT: Seasoned practitioners often make the comment, "I've been practicing for 30 years and I've never had a problem with infectious disease." Dentistry today cannot be compared with dentistry 30 years ago . . . including the challenges from infectious diseases. It's different than it was 30 years ago! The world, including the microbial world, has changed, and dentistry must adopt an efficacious infection control program as a part of patient treatment and personnel and family protection.

One of the major objections persons teaching infection control must overcome is the statement from a seasoned dental practitioner, "I've been practicing for 30 years and I've never had a problem with infectious disease . . . Why should I worry?"

Perhaps 30 years ago there may have been some truth in such a statement. However, even then there were significant threats of infectious disease in dentistry. While it is true that dentistry was less aware of such threats and that pathogens were less invasive in the wet finger environment, problems still existed. It is very dangerous for the "old guard" to compare conditions now to conditions 30 years ago. Dentistry has changed . . . the world has changed . . . and infectious diseases have changed.

What are the changes in dentistry, in the world, and in infectious diseases which are contributing to the increase of infectious diseases in the wet finger environment? First, it is important to emphasize that *THE INCREASE IN SERIOUS INFECTIOUS DISEASES IS A TRUE PERCENTAGE INCREASE AND NOT JUST AN INCREASE CAUSED BY THE GROWTH OF WORLD POPULATION,* although world population growth is one factor influencing change. Following are significant and relatively recent changes which have influenced the percentage increase of infectious diseases in dentistry.

World Travel

Anyone who has traveled by air regularly for the past 30 years recognizes the dramatic increase in world travel. Thirty years ago, the term vacation meant traveling from rural America to the "big city" for dinner, a stay in a motel, and a tour of the sights. Today, vacationing for millions of persons means traveling from the United States to Europe, Japan, Thailand, South America, New Zealand, Australia, or other distant countries formerly visited only in books. In the past few years, the beneficial exchange rate of the U.S. dollar and lowering of airfares have opened the travel door even wider for millions of Americans who were not able to visit foreign countries even a decade ago.

How does world travel effect the spread of dental

1

infectious diseases? Microbes cannot walk, they must be carried . . . in the air . . . in water . . . by fomites . . . on skin . . . on clothing . . . on hair . . . in human lungs . . . in blood . . . in saliva . . . It is arguable that AIDS would not be the serious threat to the U.S. and other parts of the world without the influence of increased world travel. This theory will be developed more fully in later chapters.

As more persons travel around the world, more microbes are being carried to and from various countries. The result is an increase of infectious diseases.

It's different than it was 30 years ago!

Immigrant Populations

Related to world travel, but effectively different, is the increased immigration of third world populations to the United States in recent years. War victims, "boat people," politically displaced Asians, Cuban exiles, Mexican nationals, and similar groups have found refuge in the United States.

Unfortunately, most immigrant groups have not had the benefit of the advanced medical treatment commonly available in the U.S.. Many persons from less advanced countries carry low-grade infectious diseases. While the systems of such persons may have adapted to the pathogens carried by them, such pathogens may be virulent to others. The result may be infection of dentists, hygienists, patients and other personnel.

Potentially infectious former immigrants are seeking dental treatment. Treating infectious persons often carries increased risk of transmitting the infection to the dental community.

It's different than it was 30 years ago!

Institutions

Federal agencies, state and local governments, and private enterprise have been very successful in creating institutions for diverse groups of persons, and much of this "institutionalizing" has occurred in the last 30-40 years. Previously, domestic institutions consisted of a few "old folks" homes, medical hospitals, tuberculosis hospitals, mental institutions, and prisons.

Today, institutions include all of the above, plus thousands of nursing homes, retirement centers, day care centers, drug abuse centers, alcohol treatment centers, weight loss centers, spas, recreational centers, psychiatric treatment centers, and many others. The United States has become one of the most "institutionalized" countries in the world.

In addition to evolving new kinds of institutions, we have also expanded the older institutions, such as hospitals and mental institutions, into institutions housing and/or treating significantly larger numbers of people. Governmental and private health insurance has contributed substantially to the growth of traditional institutions by making healthcare affordable for the domestic population.

What effect does institutionalizing people have on the spread of infectious diseases? The answer to such a question is perhaps best illustrated by the statement of Scott Holmberg, a Centers for Disease Control epidemiologist[1] when commenting on a recent epidemic of infection from salmonella-contaminated milk distributed in the Midwest. Dr. Holmberg stated:

> *. . . more and more animals [humans?] are being raised in closer quarters, and DISEASE SPREADS THAT WAY...*

Human beings are "animals" and are subject to the spread of infection that is at least partly related to the confinement in large numbers.

The New England Journal of Medicine recently published a study of the increase of tuberculosis in nursing homes,[2] a modern institution, and offered the following conclusion:

We conclude that new infection with tuberculosis is an important risk for nursing home patients. . . .

Additionally, the nosocomial rate for acquiring infectious diseases in U.S. hospitals and certain institutions is surprising to some persons. Depending upon the size and location of the hospital/institution, and whether they are private or state supported, the nosocomial rate varies from five percent to as high as 60 + percent in isolated instances. This wide variation is, in part, a result of microorganisms thriving in the institutional environment. A recent article on hospital nosocomial problems contained a comment by Dr. Lowell Levine, Professor of Public Health at Yale University, who stated:[3]

It sounds strange, but a hospital is no place for sick persons.

Persons carrying low-grade, subclinical infections acquired in one or more of our modern institutions are routinely seeking dental treatment. A high percentage of hospital personnel carry virulent *Staphylococcus aureus* in their external nares, with no obvious symptoms.

It's different than it was 30 years ago!

Lifestyle Changes

The 1960s were a period of revolutionary change in lifestyles for certain population groups. Drug abuse exploded, especially with younger groups of Americans. Communal living became popular with a small but vocal segment of society. "Coming out of the closet" by homosexuals and lesbians was encouraged. Sexual promiscuity and pornography emerged from the shadows. "Personal gratification," as long as it did not hurt anyone else, became a basic goal of living to many persons.

One result of the social revolution of the 1960s was a substantial increase in infectious disease, partly from promiscuous sex, from sharing of needles in drug abuse, and from the social phenomenon of *PEER PRESSURE.*

Numerous sociologic studies have proven that peer pressure often results in experimentation with changing lifestyles by young persons *WHO WOULD NOT HAVE EXPERIMENTED EXCEPT FOR PEER PRESSURE.*

Higher drug usage, increased sexual promiscuity, communal living, increased practice of homosexuality, and other changes in lifestyle have resulted, in large part, in an almost epidemic increase in certain infectious diseases which potentially find their way into dentistry.

It's different than it was 30 years ago!

Medical Treatment

Society equates advances in medical treatment with curing the sick and the handicapped, and certainly that is the major result of better methods of healthcare. However, there are often negative trade-offs in improved medical treatment. One very recent trade-off has been an increase in low-grade, subclinical infectious diseases as a result of the use of immunosuppressive drugs for the treatment of certain illnesses and medical problems.

Transplanting hearts and kidneys has become accepted medical treatment in much of the world. Other organ transplants and implants, including the use of artificial organs such as the mechanical heart, occupy an area of current medical experimentation. Implanting and transplanting always includes the use of *IMMUNOSUPPRESSIVE DRUGS.* Medical research has made great strides in the current use of chemotherapeutic drugs to destroy or suppress certain functions or actions of the body.

Further, researchers have recently identified possible beneficial uses of cyclosporine in the treatment of certain types of diabetes[4] and AIDS.[5] Cyclosporine is but one example of numerous *IMMUNOSUPPRESSIVE DRUGS* which act to suppress the immune system of the body. Suppressing the immune system of the body, while beneficial in certain treatment, results in the body's becoming more susceptible to infection and, in many cases, the resulting infections are low-grade and subclinical. Patients are able to lead relatively normal lives, *INCLUDING SEEKING DENTAL TREATMENT WHILE THEY ARE ALSO POTENTIALLY INFECTIOUS TO OTHERS.*

Dentistry is confronted routinely with the treatment of ambulatory, apparently "normal" patients, who are being treated with immunosuppressive drugs such as cyclosporine, corticosporine, azaathioprine, mercaptopurine, cyclophosphamide, prednisone and certain other steroids. Dental treatment carries the risk of cross-infection of the dental community with low-grade infections carried by such risk patients.

The domestic population is also living longer. Aging also results in increases in low grade infections as evidenced by a recent study of increased nosocomial infections with tuberculosis in nursing homes.[6]

It's different than it was 30 years ago!

Birth Control

Years ago, a major birth control method was the use of condoms, a form of physical barrier. With the invention of "the pill" and other chemical controls, the use of condoms became substantially reduced. Condoms actually perform two functions: 1) birth control and 2) infection control.

Direct sexual contact, increased by the reduced use of condoms, has also contributed to the increase of infectious diseases potentially finding their way into the dental environment.

It's different than it was 30 years ago!

Educational, Exchange & Self-Help Programs

Following World War II, the U.S. Government and private enterprise encouraged and financed various foreign exchange programs, including the Peace Corps, student exchange programs, agriculture teaching programs, healthcare teaching programs, technology sharing programs (such as oil exploration), and similar other programs. Depending upon the program, participants lived in advanced and emerging countries from weeks to years. Often, persons lived under substandard sanitary conditions, with the continuing threat of acquiring infectious disease.

Hundreds of thousands of Americans have participated in such programs, returning to the United States at the end of the assignment, some with chronic low-grade infections.

It's different than it was 30 years ago!

Changes in Work

Physical conditioning affects resistance to pathogenic invasion. Thirty and more years ago, many Americans were performing physical labor. Slowly, the United States has experienced a steady shift from labor-related industries to less strenuous service-related industries with the result that worker physical conditioning has often deteriorated. Physical labor has been partly replaced with recreational conditioning, such as running, jogging, and related sports activity. However, studies indicate that a significant segment of the population of the United States has become, to use the popular term, "softer." The softer the population, the less the resistance to disease.

The lessening of physical conditioning in the U.S. is resulting in a lowered resistance to disease for certain segments of society.

It's different than it was 30 years ago!

Nutritional Changes

As with a lowered resistance to infection because of reduced work-related physical conditioning, lowered nutritional levels also contribute to a reduction in resistance to infectious diseases.

In approximately the last 30 years, the U.S. has experienced an explosive growth of fast food outlets, featuring hamburgers, French fries, potato chips, ice cream, soft drinks, and similar "eat-on-the-run" items. Candy bars and soda pop have replaced apples and milk as after-school snacks. The body's nutritional needs suffer when fast foods replace a balanced diet.

It is worthy of note that the fast food industry is leading the way in protecting customers from potential cross-infection by providing disposable utensils, a protection which will hopefully become more common.

Perhaps lower levels of nutrition and a lower level of physical conditioning would be less important in the spread of infectious diseases if the other factors of world-travel, immigration, institutionalization, lifestyle changes, medical treatment, and foreign work programs were not so serious. EACH FACTOR IN THE INCREASE OF INFECTIOUS DISEASES BECOMES SYNERGISTIC AND THEREBY BECOMES MORE IMPORTANT IN THE TOTAL PICTURE.

Nutrition, too . . . it's different than it was 30 years ago!

Other less dynamic factors are also different today from those that existed 30 years ago and are also contributing to the rapid growth of infectious diseases in the United States. However, the factors listed above constitute the major contributors to the changes answering the comment, "I've never had a problem."

CONDITIONS HAVE CHANGED IN THE WORLD LAST 30 YEARS, INCLUDING IN THE WET FINGER ENVIRONMENT, AND IT IS NO LONGER REASONABLE FOR DENTAL PROFESSIONALS TO IGNORE COMPREHENSIVE INFECTION CONTROL AS A ROUTINE PART OF PATIENT TREATMENT AND PERSONNEL PROTECTION.

Summary

Seasoned dental practitioners are often heard stating, "I'm not particularly concerned about infectious diseases in dentistry." "I've been practicing 30 years, and I've never had a problem."

Such a statement may have been somewhat correct a decade or so ago. However, today, dentistry is dealing with a number of new diseases not found some years ago. Additionally, dentistry is dealing with new dynamics in the United States and in the world. World-travel, immigration, institutionalization, lifestyle changes, medical treatment, birth control, foreign self-help and work programs, changes in work, and nutritional changes are all contributing to an increase in infectious diseases in the world.

Conditions have changed in the last 30 years. Dental professionals must cope with such change by increasing efforts to control the spread of infectious disease in the dental environment.

References and Suggested Readings

1. Holmberg, S. "Millions of Us Are Probably Affected Each Year." CDC to USA TODAY, July, 1985.

2. Stead, W., *et al.* "Tuberculosis as an Endemic and Nosocomial Infection Among the Elderly in Nursing Homes." N Engl Jnl Med, 312:1483-7, June 6, 1985.

3. Levine, L. "Hospital-Contracted Infections Causing Hospital Costs to Rise." Unpublished report, Yale Univ, 1985.

4. McClaren, N. "Immune System Depressant May Fight Diabetes." Unpublished study, Univ of Fla, Coll of Med, 1985.

5. Chermann, *et al.* "Cyclosporine Used in AIDS Treatment." Public announcement, Pasteur Institute, Paris, 1985.

6. Davidson, P. "Tuberculosis: New Views of an Old Disease." N Engl Jnl Med, 312:1515-16, June 6, 1985.

CHAPTER 2

Educational Needs and Office Challenges

ABSTRACT: All members of the dental family —dentists, educators, students, hygienists, assistants, manufacturers, supplypersons, lab owners and technicians—must cooperate in the control of infectious diseases in the wet finger environment. The dental environment presents an infectious challenge because of the ways in which microbes are spread through spatters, touches, and on various instruments and surfaces.

Infection control in dentistry is undergoing dramatic change. With the publicity surrounding hepatitis, herpes, and AIDS, dentists, dental auxiliaries, laboratory personnel and consumers are becoming acutely aware that the dental environment is a potential source of one or more of these diseases. As it has been shown that some of these diseases can be spread in dental offices and laboratories, the concern has been raised as to what new diseases may also infect dental personnel and patients in the future.

A minimal concern for infection control in dentistry for many years has left dental personnel vulnerable to many infections in the population that are transmissible in *SALIVA* and *BLOOD*. A high exposure to hepatitis B has been clearly demonstrated.[1] AIDS has dramatically raised dental awareness that other new diseases may challenge dentistry in the future. Microbiologists are carefully observing certain of the neurologic "slow viruses," questioning whether they may begin challenging the dental environment.[2]

The control of dental infectious diseases is not the obligation of any single dental group. Dentists, educators, students, hygienists, assistants, "outer office" staff, manufacturers, supply persons, laboratory owners, and technicians, in short all dental healthcare personnel, must cooperate if the spread of infections through dental facilities is to be prevented. It is very important to realize that on any single day *EACH ONE OF THESE INDIVIDUALS MAY BE CONFRONTED WITH AN INFECTIOUS DISEASE.*

It is not necessary to be engaged in the direct treatment of patients to be exposed to infection. A supply person talking to a dentist or an assistant in the office may be the victim. Laboratory personnel, whether from a private or commercial "lab," may be exposed during pick-up and delivery to the office and through the handling of contaminated impressions, models, and appliances.

What can be done to correct the deficiencies of the past and to control the infection problems of the future? FIRST, THE AWARENESS LEVEL OF EVERYONE CONNECTED WITH DENTISTRY MUST BE RAISED. THE PROBLEM MUST BE UNDERSTOOD! SECOND, THERE MUST BE A COOPERATIVE EFFORT TO RESPECT THE RIGHTS TO THE PREVENTION OF INFECTION IN ALL PERSONS—

WHETHER PATIENTS, DENTISTS, AUXI-LIARIES, SUPPLY PERSONS OR LABORA-TORY PERSONNEL. In all dental disciplines, control procedures must be adopted and practiced which will act to reduce the possibility of exposure to infection.

Educational Needs

Historically, dental schools have not taught infection control with the same emphasis as they have taught restorative procedures. The teaching of practical office infection control has been relegated to a lower priority. Schools have been more concerned with the establishment of procedures for the sterilization of instruments in a central, presumably well-controlled, environment by salaried employees. The basic assumption has been that only in this way can schools protect patients and students from infection. The result of the centralized method of sterilization is that dental students have not learned an effective infection control program which could be transferred directly from their schools to their offices. This educational philosophy has limited students to minimal hands-on experience, and the newly-graduated dentist has been left deficient in infection control expertise.

At a meeting in March, 1985, the House of Delegates of the American Association of Dental Schools adopted a resolution recommending the use of barriers (gloves, masks, eyeglasses, etc.) in dental school clinics.

Whereas schools have relegated infection control to a lower priority in the past, there presently appears to be a sincere and dedicated effort to prepare dental students for the infectious disease challenges they will face in practice after graduation. Change will not come rapidly, but it will come.

Presently, the majority of students graduating from dental schools are still not prepared for the practical challenges of wet finger infection control. As a result of many schools' emphasis on central sterilization with minimal attention to practical office situations, typically the recently graduated dentist faced with infection control has three alternatives: 1) to accept advice from older practitioners whose infection procedures may be minimal and outdated, 2) to accept advice from dental supply personnel who may lack the necessary education and experience to serve as consultants on such a vital subject, or 3) to rely on the knowledge a "trained" assistant gained in previous practices.

It must be recognized that auxiliaries are often "left on their own" by dentist employers. They may be left to their own resources to gather infection control information, and, even though they may be highly motivated, they may not be able to formulate a complete program. Accordingly, new graduates must be able to assess the knowledge of their axuliaries.

Well-intentioned suppliers may recommend products, not systems, and they are occasionally influenced in their recommendations by considerations other than product efficacy and suitability. However, because of the often close relationship between dental suppliers and dental offices, suppliers can sometimes be a good resource in the adoption and refinement of an infection control program. Progressive suppliers are in a good position to pre-screen new products for recommendation to dental personnel.

The knowledge of previously "trained" dental assistants is only as complete as their previous education or experience. Newly-graduated dentists often are not able to judge the depth nor correctness of that knowledge.

Infection control often becomes a "do-it-your-self-project" in which there are many opinions from various advisers, but there are few all-around experts. Dentists and dental personnel have the professional and legal obligation and the personal responsibility to become knowledgeable in infection control procedures and products in order to lead the way in establishing and implementing effective control programs for the prevention of infection in their patients and their fellow workers.

Office Challenges

Before considering the various components of an infection control program, one must understand the exposure to infection that is inherent in an average dental procedure. A practitioner in a general dental office serves from ten to thirty patients each day who require examinations, emergency treatment, and "drop-in service." This patient load usually includes many types and ages of people from different economic conditions — the old and the young, the rich and the poor. Their personal habits, daily activities, and types of work vary. Consequently, they have varying degrees of exposure to infection. Recently, these problems have been compounded by the increase in certain groups of immigrants, such as "boat people" from Southeast Asia, who may be highly infectious. All of these variables are funneled into a dental chair in a working treatment area approximately 120 square feet in size, where a dentist and one or two assistants are in close proximity for up to an hour or more. All of the participants in this potentially infective exercise are exposed to the microbes that result from talking, coughing, sneezing, or touching, and to additional microbes spread during invasive dental procedures.

An illustration of the potential infective problems may be seen in this description of a hypothetical dental treatment. After the patient is seated, the assistant takes several X-rays and the "wet finger" process begins as saliva is spread from the patient's mouth to the X-ray exposure button and the X-ray head. The dentist injects an anesthetic and prepares to do a restoration. Next, the dentist uses a drill rotating at several hundred thousand revolutions per minute, thereby creating an aerosol of water, saliva and blood extending several feet around the patient's mouth. The severity of this aerosol is best demonstrated by examining glasses worn by dental personnel during a drilling procedure. The glasses will be covered with literally hundreds of minute spatters and droplets.

The dentist places the contaminated drill in the handpiece holder, takes an instrument from the bracket table or set-up tray, of course with "wet fingers," and re-enters the mouth. The assistant washes the cavity with a jet of water from the syringe, with resultant splashes of saliva, water, and blood, which the assistant evacuates from the mouth by grasping the high volume evacuation holder and rotating the tip between the patient's tongue and cheek.

The dentist moves the patient's head and readjusts the light — again with "wet fingers." The cavity preparation is completed, and the dentist presses a matrix retainer, band, and wedge into place. The assistant washes blood and saliva away with a jet of water from the three-way syringe and evacuates the mixture with the high volume evacuation (HVE). The dentist dries the cavity with a blast of air and places a liner, while the assistant mixes the amalgam in the amalgamator, loaded and turned on with "wet fingers." The dentist's hands move to and from the bracket table with increasing numbers of instruments. He inserts several cotton rolls and removes the matrix retainer, band, and wedge. After the washing and evacuating of the mouth, the patient empties water, saliva, excess amalgam, and blood into the cuspidor bowl. Since one-half of the lower jaw is anesthetized, the patient misses the center of the bowl, and debris splashes onto the surrounding equipment, the floor, and the wall, which has already been contaminated by sprays and splashes from the handpiece and air/water syringe.

The dentist gives the patient final instructions, makes notes on the patient records, without washing the hands, and leaves, while the assistant pushes appropriate buttons on the chair so that the patient may exit. The chair had been adjusted several times during the procedure — necessarily with "wet fingers." By the time the patient is gone, much of the treatment area, from instruments to patient records, has become contaminated; furthermore, everyone from the dentist to an occasional observer such as a dental supply representative, has been exposed to concentrations of potential pathogens. This scenario is repeated many times each day.

Dr. James Crawford, Professor of Microbiology at the University of North Carolina Dental School, originated a unique series of slides to illustrate some of the sepsis that results in cross-contamination in the wet finger environment. Dr. Crawford simulated saliva with a diluted commercial solution with red poster paint. He then instructed a hygienist in the school dental clinic to perform a prophylaxis on a mannikin-patient. The resulting red splashes on patient, practitioner, and chairside staff are most alarming. Each "red spot" illustrates a potential cross-infection area.

Bacterilogic studies of similar surfaces of dental units and equipment as those illustrated in the Saliva Were Red series verified actual microbial contamination during patient treatment.[3]

Initially, it may seem that infection control is impossible in such a septic environment. However, REASONABLY ACCURATE IDENTIFICATION OF RISK CATEGORIES, OBSERVING CAREFUL PRECAUTIONS, AND PRACTICING EFFECTIVE CONTROL PROCEDURES CAN KEEP INFECTIOUS MICROORGANISMS WITHIN THE MANAGEABLE LIMITS OF THE BODY'S RESISTANCE TO DISEASE, THEREBY MINIMIZING CONTAMINATION AND CROSS-INFECTION OF THE DENTAL FAMILY.

Summary

Infectious diseases are increasing in the world and in the United States. The awareness of such problems must be raised in all dental professionals, auxiliaries, and others contacting the dental environment to assure a coordinated effort directed toward controlling cross-infection in dentistry.

Dental educators and dental practitioners are all confronted with infection control challenges. One answer to such challenges is for dental practitioners to learn to identify profiles of Routine, Risk and High Risk patients.

References and Suggested Readings

1. Cottone, J. "Hepatitis B Virus Infection in the Dental Profession." JADA 110:617-21, Apr, 1985.

2. Crawford, J. Personal communication, Univ of NC, 1985.

3. Crawford, J. "If Saliva Were Red." Slide presentation, Univ of NC, 1979.

Understanding the Basics

ABSTRACT: It is necessary to understand terminology, microbial life, modes and routes of transmission, cross-contamination, and other basics to fully comprehend the problems of dental infectious diseases.

Before proceeding further, a thorough understanding of certain basics is necessary. The following information is not intended as a course in basic microbiology. It is impossible to present more than the rudiments in these few pages; therefore, it is strongly urged that those readers who do not process such information secure basic microbiology textbooks for a more in-depth review. Infection control is a changing, evolving field. Practitioners and personnel can better cope with change if they have a reasonable comprehension of biological terms and bodily functions.

Definitions

The following definitions will be useful in understanding the basics of infection control and in comprehending content of the other chapters.

1. *Acute*—Sharp and severe. Quick, critical, crucial.
2. *Animal*—Any living thing that is not a plant.
3. *Animate*—To give life. Alive.
4. *Antimicrobial*—Working against microbes, as in antimicrobial soap.
5. *Aseptic*—The same as sterile. Characterized by total absence of life.
6. *Autogenous or endogenous infection*—Infection originating from within one's own body.
7. *Biological*-Of plant and animal life.
8. *Carrier*—A person who harbors and disseminates a micro-organism capable of causing disease in another person. A carrier commonly has a subclinical case of the disease, thus appearing and feeling well.
9. *Catalyze*—Causing or speeding an action or reaction.
10. *Chemotherapy*—Treatment of a disease or infection with chemicals, without harming the host.
11. *Chronic*—Long-lasting, lingering, continuous.
12. *Coagulate*—Change from liquid to thickened mass.
13. *Cross-contamination*—Contamination passed from one person or inanimate object to another.
14. *Cross-infection*—Infection passed from one person to another.

15. *Disease* — Interruption by an infective agent in the normal performance of the vital functions of a plant or animal.
16. *Disinfection* — Destruction of most micro-organisms, but not necessarily all, especially not highly resistant forms such as spores.
17. *Exogenous infection* — Infection originating from an external source.
18. *Exudate* — Oozing, usually of a clear liquid from a sore, lesion, or body opening.
19. *Host* — A plant or animal having a parasite (micro-organism) habitually living on or in it.
20. *Immune* — Protected from disease by body's defenses.
21. *Immunosuppressive* — A drug or agent that retards or suppresses the natural immune system of the body.
22. *Inanimate* — Without life.
23. *Infection* — Establishment of a microorganism on or in a host.
24. *Infectious disease* — A harmful infection.
25. *Inorganic* — Not having the structure of living things. Not produced by animal or plant activities.
26. *Lifestyle* — Circumstances and environment which govern an individual life; conditions of housing, recreation, sexual activity, medical care, etc., must be considered.
27. *Micro-organism, microbe* — Animals or plants which can be seen only through a microscope.
28. *Mode of transmission* — Method, device, or vehicle by which microbes are transmitted from one place or person to another place or person.
29. *Morbidity* — The proportion of sickness in a certain group or locality.
30. *Mortality* — Frequency of death.
31. *Nosocomial* — Having to do with a hospital; colloquially used to describe infections acquired in hospitals or other institutions.
32. *Opportunistic pathogens* — Microorganisms which are normally not harmful but may become pathogenic when there is a break in the body's defenses, as might occur in the case of an immune suppressed patient.
33. *Organic* — Of the bodily organs. Produced by animal or plant activities, containing carbon.
34. *Pathogenic* — Disease producing.
35. *Plant* — A member of the vegetable kingdom; not animal; usually distinguished from animal by absence of locomotion and special organs of sensation and digestion, and by the power of living wholly upon inorganic substances.
36. *Regulatory agency* — Governmental body which reviews and implements/enforces certains laws/guidelines.
37. *Resistance* — Ability of the body to overcome invading pathogens and prevent harmful infection. "Resist" infection.
38. *Risk patient* — An individual who, because of physical condition, medical treatment, occupation, lifestyle, age, or other circumstance, may be carrying/transmitting pathogenic micro-organisms.
39. *Route of transmission* — Portal, opening or vehicle through which or by which microbes enter or are carried to the body.
40. *Sanitize* — To make as clean as possible but not to disinfect.
41. *Septic* — Contaminated, infected, or putrified.
42. *Serology* — Study of the use of serums in diagnosing, curing, or preventing disease.
43. *Serum* — Clear, watery part of the blood that separates from the clot when blood coagulates.
44. *Spore forms* — Inactive form of microorganisms, more highly resistant to disinfection or sterilization than are vegetative forms.
45. *Sterilization* — Total destruction of all life.
46. *Subclinical (low-grade) infection* — An infection without apparent symptoms. Infected persons are usually ambulatory and are able to carry on a relatively normal life.
47. *Surgical scrub* — The process of cleaning hands, arms, and skin with meticulous care, utilizing an antimicrobial soap, brush, and antimicrobial rinse.
48. *Synergistic* — An action producing a greater effect than the sum of the individual actions; colloquially $1 + 1 = 3$.
49. *Vegetative forms* — Active microorganisms, less resistant to disinfection or sterilization.

50. *Virulence* — The relative ease with which a microorganism breaks down the body's defenses.
51. *Virus forms* — Sub-microscopic, potentially infective particles composed of protein and nucleic acid.

Microbial Life

The human body is engineered to be an ideal host for the growth of microorganisms. Nutrition is supplied from blood, serum, decayed food, and other sources, and the ideal normal body temperature of 98.6 degrees Fahrenheit encourages rapid growth. Microbial life is desirable and necessary in the human life cycle. Without beneficial microbes to aid, for example in the digestion of food, life would change substantially, perhaps even cease. Certainly life would be more difficult. Danger is present only when opportunistic/foreign microbes infect the body.

Infection control requires a basic working knowledge of microbiology, a term which is somewhat self-explanatory — *micro* meaning tiny, and *biology* meaning the study of physical life. Microbiology then is the study of microorganisms and all factors influencing the life, growth, evolution, function, and death of such organisms.

There are hundreds of types of microbes, but for our purposes several broad groups are important: the *NON-PATHOGENIC,* the *OPPORTUNISTIC* and *PATHOGENIC,* and those that are *RESISTANT* and *LESS RESISTANT* to disinfection or sterilization.

Pathogenic, or disease-producing, microbes are the villains of infection and fortunately are less abundant than beneficial or non-pathogenic microbes. Some pathogens become merely aggravations, such as the common cold, while others can be deadly, such as with hepatitis B or tuberculosis. During the treatment of patients, dental personnel are exposed to multiple kinds of microorganisms of varying pathogenicity.

Opportunistic microbes are those microorganisms that take advantage of some compromise in a host to initiate infection. When an unusual circumstance occurs, such as reduced resistance by the host, the opportunistic microbe can then become pathogenic. A good example of opportunistic microbes may be seen in certain yeasts of the candida group. These microbes exist in substantial numbers in much of everyday life. They remain harmless until lowering of the resistance of the host occurs, as with a patient on immunosuppressive drug therapy, at which time the microbes may create serious infection of the mucous membrane, mouth, throat, vagina, or similar tissues.

Lay persons often think that the deadlier microbes are the more difficult to kill. Such is not always the case. *The virulence, or deadliness, of microbes is not necessarily related to the difficulty with which the microbes are destroyed.* Some highly threatening forms, such as the AIDS virus, are relatively easy to destroy with an effective disinfectant, such as an iodophor, simply by leaving a film of the moist disinfectant on a surface where the virus is likely to exist. On the other hand, bacterial spores, some of which may be harmless by themselves, are destroyed only by an effective sterilizer. This difference in vulnerability is important because disinfection is very important in practical infection control. If most pathogens were highly resistant to eradication and were susceptible only to sterilants, disinfection would be relatively useless. Disinfection is the only practical method of microbial control available for the treatment of most equipment, surfaces, cabinets, floors, and other large items.

The level of resistance to kill is also important in microbiological testing for the effectiveness of sterilization procedures.

Since microbial life can be seen only through a microscope, infection control is a science of "faith." Except for the use of biological monitors, the results of infection control procedures are seldom seen in the dental environment. This lack of visibility makes the choice of procedures and products extremely important. If the procedures or the products do

13

not perform as claimed, infection may result, and patients and dental staff will pay the price. When accepting advice or instruction on infection control, one should know the expertise of the teacher. When purchasing infection control products, one should study reliable written *INDEPENDENT* scientific data from accepted publications and information supporting the claims being made, and one should use only "legal" products as discussed in Chapter 8.

It is very beneficial for infection control personnel to take courses in basic microbiology. Some microbiology courses are designed to teach the classifications, shapes, sizes, mobility, cellular structure, and other physical characteristics of microbes. However, courses are less useful in infection control than courses designed to give a working knowledge of the world of microbes and their interface with the visible world, such as those taught in health sciences related programs. For home study purposes, the microbiology department of a university can recommend textbooks. Several useful texts are included in the suggested readings.[1]

Modes and Routes of Transmission

Certain body systems provide natural resistance to microbial invasion. For example, the oral cavity is lined with mucosal tissue which serves to protect the body from foreign substances. Similar tissues line the entire digestive system. It is only when the mucosa is broken or cut, for example with a dental bur, that the body is exposed to infection by invasion through this body system.

Penetrating the oral mucosa with an instrument, thereby admitting foreign microbes into the blood stream, is one example of the various modes of pathogenic transmission. Other modes include saliva, nasal discharge, semen, hands, hair, vaginal secretions, breast milk, clothing, dust, water, body waste, and nearly every vehicle onto which a microbe may become attached. Once the microbes have been transported to a host, they must enter the body through a suitable route of transmission of infection to begin the growth phase of the infective process, in which the microbes multiply and spread to susceptible parts of the body.

The skin, mucosa and other resistive coverings and linings of the body and its organs are designed to prevent microbial invasion. However, the natural body openings are common routes of transmission. For example, inhaling opens a direct path from the mouth or nose to the lungs and thereby to the blood system. The nose is a portal of entry to the easily infected sinuses, and the nose also allows infective entry to the middle ear and beyond if the ear drum is ruptured. The genital openings invite entry to many pathogens.

When invading microbes appear, the body resists infection by activating natural defense processes. An elevated temperature (fever) helps control microbial growth by making the body an uncomfortable host. Certain body cells (macrophages) attempt to capture and destroy invaders through a process called phagocytosis. Then, the body tissues try to wall off the invaders in localized areas (abscesses) to give the other body processes time to come to the defense of the host. Body fluids attempt to wash the invaders away, as with the "sniffles" of the common cold. A general feeling of tiredness (malaise) forces the infected person to rest and thereby to conserve strength which can then be used to fight the infection. All of these and other defenses are helpful, but the more virulent diseases are sometimes too strong to be overcome, especially in the elderly, the infirm, and the compromised patient.

Stated as an equation, infection may be defined thus:

$$Infection = \frac{Virulence \times Number\ of\ microbes}{Resistance\ of\ host}$$

The dental office can do little about the virulence of the organisms, because it is seldom known which organisms are present. Dentists may influence the resistance of the host before treatment in some cases by prescribing better nutrition, exercise, rest and other sensible "self-help" programs. In certain instances, it may be desirable to postpone all but emergency dental care until the resistance of the host is enhanced.

THE DENTAL OFFICE CAN REASONABLY REDUCE THE NUMBER OF ORGANISMS ON INSTRUMENTS, SURFACES, AND OTHER AREAS OF THE DENTAL ENVIRONMENT.

The dental office must help to reduce to an absolute minimum the number of microbes in the environment, on personnel, on equipment, on instruments, and on other areas of patient contact. The number of microbes is the one part of the equation which can be controlled by office procedures.

ONE GOAL OF AN INFECTION CONTROL PROGRAM IS TO REDUCE THE NUMBER OF AVAILABLE PATHOGENIC MICROBES TO A LEVEL WHERE THE NORMAL RESISTANCE MECHANISMS OF THE BODY MAY PREVENT INFECTION.

Autogenous Infection

Dental personnel are obligated to help control autogenous infections, for example, by: a) preventing post-treatment, potentially life-threatening infections caused by significant amounts of bacterial plaque and calculus from being introduced into tissues during extractions and other procedures that penetrate tissue; and b) through the administration of prophylactic antibiotic treatment to prevent bacterial growth on damaged heart valves in a patient who has experienced rheumatic heart disease. An equally important infection control obligation of the dental office is the prevention of cross-contamination, and thus the prevention of cross-infection. The carrier mode of some diseases makes infection acquired as a result of cross-contamination often more serious than that of a self-induced infection.

Cross-Contamination

Cross-contamination, which may lead to cross-infection, may occur in a number of ways. A casual sneeze or a cough can spray contaminated saliva or airborne pathogenic microbes. Touching surfaces which have been contaminated with pathogens is another method.[2] Such casual contact, while dangerous, is not the major source of dental infective transmission from patient to personnel, from personnel to personnel, or from personnel to patients. Potentially infective pathogens are found in the highest concentrations in blood and saliva; therefore, any procedure involving these fluids carries the most danger to patients and staff. As previously described, cuts or breaks in the skin or mucosa offer a direct route for pathogens to the blood stream, allowing them to by-pass certain of the body's resistance systems.

A typical example of cross-contamination involves a carrier patient, harboring a disease such as hepatitis B, and a dental assistant. The dental assistant nicks her finger with the tip of an explorer as she is scrubbing instruments with her bare hands in preparation for sterilization. The assistant returns to the treatment area without wearing gloves, and she assists the dentist by evacuating saliva and blood from the patient's mouth. Hepatitis viruses from the patient's saliva enter the assistant's blood stream through the nicked finger with the result of a crossing, or cross-contamination, from the patient to the assistant. This same transmission can occur from or to various persons in and out of the office. The ultimate result of cross-contamination is an unending cycle.

The question is occasionally asked, "Are dental offices really a serious source of cross-contamination, and, if so, how often?" Ohio State University did an interesting study in 1980 to determine if cross-contamination in a dental hygiene clinic was a significant problem. The study[3] was carefully designed to repeat daily procedures as routinely performed in the clinic. The protocol provided a realistic way to trace microorganisms from 20 patients' mouths to hygienists' hands, chair switches, and sink

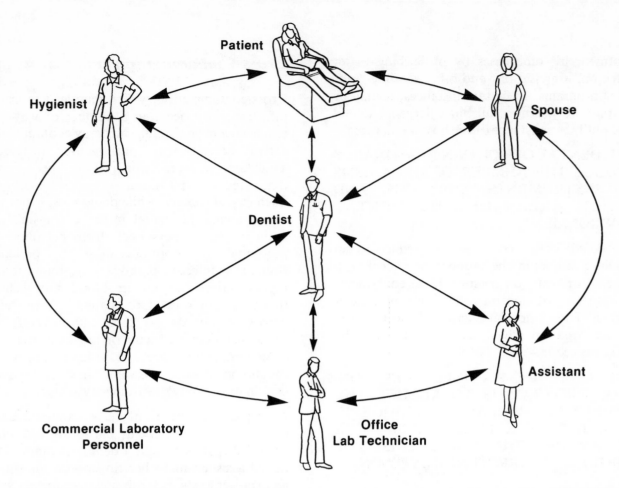

Patient

Hygienist

Spouse

Dentist

Commercial Laboratory
Personnel

Office
Lab Technician

Assistant

faucets. Results concluded that there was a significant amount of cross-contamination in the clinic. Potentially pathogenic organisms were routinely transferred from the patients' mouths to the fingers of the dental hygiene students, and then to the switches on the dental chair and to the handles of the sink. These organisms may then be transferred from the inanimate objects to the next patient. Adding additional credibility to this study is a recent study showing that foreign blood was found under the fingernails of healthcare workers five days after treating patients.[4]

Historically, many of the reasons for practicing prevention of dental cross-contamination centered on the need to protect patients from infection. There were often fewer concerns about the dangers that dentists and staff would acquire infection from patients. Beginning with the recognition of the dangers of hepatitis B and accelerating with recent concerns of potential infection of personnel with herpes and AIDS, health personnel are becoming increasingly

concerned with the dangers of treating infected patients. It is essential that dental offices, hospitals, and hospital dental services review their infection control procedures so that state-of-the-art practices may be utilized for maximal protection of personnel.

ANOTHER GOAL OF AN INFECTION CONTROL PROGRAM IS TO BREAK THE CIRCLE OF INFECTION AND ELIMINATE CROSS-CONTAMINATION.

AIDS has received dramatic and continuous media attention recently as even public figures have admitted to being infected with the disease. One result of the media coverage has been to alarm some dental personnel who do not understand the important facts of the disease and who do not understand the basics of efficacious infection control.

As a result of fear of the unknown, it is becoming increasingly difficult for AIDS patients to obtain dental care. One area of the country has found it necessary to establish a private clinic, staffed with volunteer dental personnel, to provide dental care to AIDS patients.[5]

As of the date of this publication, only approximately 40,000 persons have been identified in the U.S. as having Stage 3 AIDS. Because of this relatively small number, many persons in dentistry perceive that they are able to minimize exposure to the disease by refusing to treat infected patients. However, refusing to treat infected persons will become increasingly more difficult as the AIDS epidemic grows and as it becomes more pervasive in our society. Even-

tually, a substantial segment of dentistry must learn to treat AIDS patients and patients infected with other serious diseases.

It was estimated in 1986 by Dr. James Curran of the Centers for Disease Control and by other authorities that the number of persons then infected with the AIDS virus was approximately 1,750,000[6] and that the number was growing daily. Present evidence indicates that more than two million are undiagnosed and infected with AIDS. Such persons may be more contagious than individuals with Classical (Stage 3) AIDS. The same scenario is present with hepatitis B.

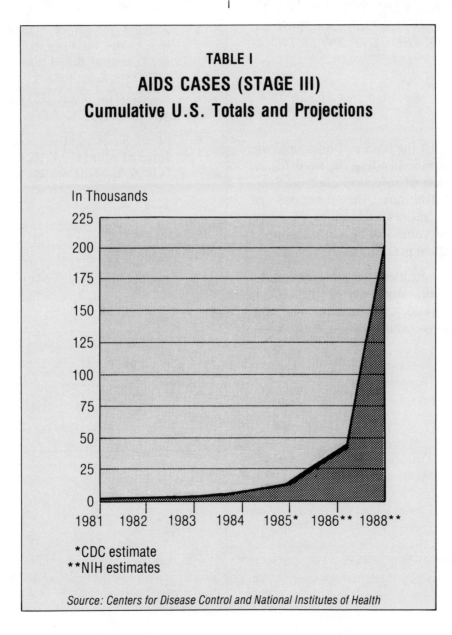

TABLE I

AIDS CASES (STAGE III)
Cumulative U.S. Totals and Projections

In Thousands

*CDC estimate
**NIH estimates

Source: Centers for Disease Control and National Institutes of Health

Table 1 illustrates the predicted growth of Stage 3 AIDS through 1988, according to the CDC and the U.S. Public Health Service. If Dr. Curran and other noted researchers are correct in predicting that the AIDS virus has spread to nearly two million Americans, efforts by dentists to evade the virus by refusing to treat certain patients are ultimately bound to fail.

A MORE REASONABLE APPROACH TO CONTROLLING EXPOSURE TO AIDS AND OTHER INFECTIOUS DISEASES IS TO IMPLEMENT INFECTION CONTROL PROCEDURES WHICH EFFECTIVELY MINIMIZE THE POSSIBILITY THAT PATIENTS . . . AND THE DENTAL FAMILY . . . WILL ACQUIRE ANY INFECTIOUS DISEASE.

Summary

An understanding of the basics of microbial life is necessary for comprehending the need for an efficacious program of infection control. Staff understanding definitions, the functions of microbes, and the modes and routes of transmission of such microbes will be better equipped to institute and repeat procedures.

Microorganisms routinely contaminate the dental environment, and dental personnel, unless very careful and very conscientious, may contribute to cross-contamination and cross-infection.

References and Suggested Readings

1. Morello, J., Mizer, H., and Wilson, M. MICROBIOLOGY IN PATIENT CARE (4th Ed, McMillan, New York, 1984).

   Tortora, G., Funk, Burdell, and Case. MICROBIOLOGY, AN INTRODUCTION (Benjamin/Cummins Pub, Menlo Park, CA, 1982).

2. Miller, C. "The Case for Gloves." Dent Asepsis Rvw, 4:9:1, Sept, 1983.

3. Autio, Rosen, *et al.* "Studies on Cross-contamination in the Dental Chair." JADA, Mar, 1980.

4. Allen, A., Organ, R. "Occult Blood Accumulation Under the Fingernails: A Mechanism for the Spread of Blood-borne Infection." JADA, 105:455-9, Sept, 1982.

5. Schaefer, M. Personal communication, Univ of So Cal, 1985.

6. Sivak, S., *et al.* "Estimated Number of Adults Infected with HTLV-III in the United States." N Engl Jnl Med, Nov 21, 1985.

Chapter Three
REVIEW EXERCISES

Date _____Name_____

Circle the letters of the terms which most closely approximate the answers. There may be one or more than one correct answer. If you circle D, indicate the other answer or answers, if known.

1. The most resistant microorganisms are:

   A. vegetative

   B. pathogens

   C. spores

   D. other_____

2. Disease producing microorganisms are:

   A. pathogens

   B. carriers

   C. spores

   D. other_____

3. The total destruction of all life is:

   A. disinfection

   B. infection

   C. sterilization

   D. other_____

4. The ease with which microbes break down the body's defenses is:

   A. infection

   B. virulence

   C. disease

   D. other_____

5. The process of passing infection from one person to another is:

   A. cross-infection

   B. endogenous infection

   C. carrier

   D. other_____

6. Aseptic is the same as:

   A. septic

   B. sanitary

   C. sterilized

   D. other_____

7. Viruses are:

   A. vegetative forms

   B. infective particles

   C. spore forms

   D. other_____

8. Disease producing microbes are:

   A. easy to kill

   B. hard to kill

   C. pathogenic

   D. other_____

9. The hepatitis B virus is:

   A. not too serious

   B. a major dental threat

   C. indigenous to Australia

   D. other_____

10. Infection control procedures are:

    A. an exact science

    B. a science of faith

    C. highly visible

    D. other_____

11. Courses in microbiology most useful in infection control teach:

    A. microbial structure

    B. physical facts of microbes

    C. microbial interface with the visible world

    D. other_____

12. Natural resistance to microbial invasion is found in:

    A. the oral cavity

    B. all healthy body systems

    C. the oral mucosa

    D. other_____

13. Modes of transmission include:

    A. blood

    B. saliva

    C. semen

    D. other_____

14. The most dangerous instrument in the dental office in terms of infection control is:

    A. scalpel   B. extraction forcep   C. dental bur

    D. other_____

15. The most difficult protective covering to cut is:

    A. skin   B. mucosa   C. gingiva

    D. other_____

16. Natural defense mechanisms of the body include:

    A. fever   B. abscesses   C. malaise

    D. other_____

17. The goal of an effective infection control program is:

    A. to get new patients   B. to sterilize everything C. to reduce the number of
                                                              microbes in the environment

    D. other_____

18. Professional offices are obligated to:

    A. treat the needy   B. prevent cross-contamination C. prevent infection

    D. other_____

19. Potentially infective pathogens are found in highest concentrations:

    A. on skin   B. in blood   C. in saliva

    D. other_____

20. Cross-contamination is:

    A. only a medical   B. a "hidden" disease   C. a venereal disease
       problem

    D. other_____

NOTE: Answers to the review exercises appear in the back of this book.

Diseases of Special Concern

ABSTRACT: A relatively large number of pathogenic micro-organisms may frequently be carried into and out of dental offices by patients and personnel. Some of the diseases are visible to the trained eye, and some are not.

Emerging "new" diseases, such as hepatitis (and AIDS), present a special problem if effective infection control procedures are not practiced by the dentist and staff.

Inadequate procedures may have devastating effect on health, income, and prevention of malpractice.

Dental personnel are potentially exposed to a surprisingly large number of serious diseases, some of which may cause death.

Experienced dentists sometimes feel that concern about infection is exaggerated because they "have never been bothered with serious disease problems." The fallacy in such a statement is that the dentist or his staff may never know if they have caused an infection, since many carriers are not aware of their problems. Many practitioners do not realize the number of pathogens that are regularly carried to and from their offices.

When health practitioners choose careers in the health sciences, they assume a moral and legal obligation to protect patients. That obligation must be fulfilled. Dentistry must increasingly recognize the importance of its role in limiting the spread of disease.

Table 2 on the following page lists the major diseases which confront dental offices.

Classifying Dental Diseases

For purposes of simplification, dental diseases may be classified as CLINICAL (VISIBLE), SUB-CLINICAL (INVISIBLE), and EMERGING (NEW). Infection control procedures for all three categories are the same, but motivation for personnel to use special precautions may depend upon the physical characteristics of the diseases and the ease with which they can be identified.

Clinical (Visible) Diseases

Dental personnel are potentially exposed to a number of clinical diseases. Some of the diseases, such as syphilis and herpes, are identifiable by lesions or other apparent symptoms. Following are some examples of clinical diseases:

Syphilis	Measles
Gonorrhea	Chicken pox
Herpes simplex	Mumps

It is usual for dental personnel to react to the visible signs of these diseases by protecting

23

TABLE 2
SERIOUS INFECTIOUS DISEASES FOUND IN DENTISTRY

Disease	Agent	Route Of Transmission	Incubation Period	Potential Complications
Acquired Immune Deficiency Syndrome (AIDS)	Virus	Sexual contact, blood, other body fluids(?)	Lifetime(?)	Death
Chicken Pox	Virus	Saliva, blood, droplets	10-21 days	Conjunctivitis, shingles, Encephalitis
Common Cold	Virus	Saliva, blood, droplets	48-72 hours	Temporary disability
Cytomegalovirus	Virus	Oral	2-8 weeks	Birth defects, death
Gonorrhea	Bacteria	Sexual contact	1-7 days	Arthritis, female sterility, infant blindness
Hepatitis A	Virus	Oral, fecal	2-7 weeks	Disability
Hepatitis B	Virus	Saliva, blood, droplets	6 weeks-6 months	Chronic disability, carrier mode death
Hepatitis (non-A, non-B)	Virus	Saliva, blood, droplets	6 weeks-5 months	Chronic disability, death
Hepatitis Delta	"Piggy back" virus	Blood, other routes under investigation	Not known	Death, chronic carrier
Hepetic Conjunctivitis	Virus	Saliva, blood, droplets	6-10 weeks	Potential blindness
Herpes Simplex II	Virus	Sexual contact, possible saliva, blood	Up to 2 weeks Also latent	Painful lesions, disability, death in children
Herpetic Whitlow	Virus	Saliva, blood, droplets	2-12 days. Also latent	Extreme pain, disability
Infectious Mononucleosis	Virus	Saliva, blood, droplets	4-7 weeks	Temporary disability
Influenza	Virus	Saliva, droplets	1-3 days	Death
Legionellosis	Bacteria	Respiratory	2-10 days	Death
Measles (German)	Virus	Saliva, nasal, droplets	9-11 days	Congenital defects, infant death
Measles (Rubeola)	Virus	Saliva, nasal, droplets	9-11 days	Temporary disability, encephalitis
Mumps (men)	Virus	Respiratory	14-25 days	Temporary disability, sterility
Pneumonia	Bacteria, Virus	Respiratory, blood blood	Varies with organism	Death
Staphyloccus Infections	Bacteria	Saliva, droplets, nosocomial	4-10 days	Skin lesions, osteomyelitis, death
Streptococcus Infections	Bacteria	Saliva, blood, droplets	1-3 days	Rheumatic heart, kidney problems, death
Syphilis	Bacteria	Sexual contact, congenital	2-12 weeks	Central nervous damage, death
Tetanus	Bacteria	Open wound	7-10 days	Disability, death
Tuberculosis	Bacteria	Saliva, droplets	Up to 6 months Also latent	Disability, death

themselves and others from cross-contamination.

Certain diseases, such as measles, mumps, and chicken pox, may not seem potentially serious. Yet such "normal" infections can be very serious to dentists and staff, with sequelae such as herpes zoster and shingles.

Some years ago the author was rushing to complete some last minute office details in preparation for a vacation when a five-year-old male child was brought in for an emergency. The mother said the child had not felt well for a few days and that his mouth "bothered" him. In the haste of the last minute treatment, precautions were not taken to protect staff from what should have been recognized as a child with a systemic infection. No one wore a mask or gloves or took other normally routine precautions.

The author and his family proceeded on the vacation, and a few days later the author began developing increasingly uncomfortable symptoms, and it became necessary to seek hospital treatment. After several days of tests, chicken pox was diagnosed and complete disability continued for weeks.

The author was finally released from the hospital and was allowed to return home for weeks of convalescence. The attending physician commented on the seriousness of childhood diseases in adults. Death is not unheard of in such cases.

The moral to the story is that the treatment of the child patient should have been postponed, both for the comfort of the child and for the protection of the staff. If treatment had been necessary, effective infection control procedures would probably have prevented infection of the author and the subsequent serious complications, including loss of income, large medical and hospital expenses, and loss of jealously guarded vacation time.

Sub-Clinical (Invisible) Diseases

Sub-clinical diseases seldom give staff pre-warning of a potential infection because such diseases do not show visible lesions, rash, or other obvious evidence. Symptoms may be low-grade and are sometimes not recognized even by the infected. Following are some examples of sub-clinical diseases:

Creutzfeld Jakob Disease
Hepatitis (various strains)
Infectious mononucleosis
Influenza
Pneumonia
Tuberculosis

Of course, sub-clinical diseases are much more serious because there are fewer warning signals and, therefore, personnel may not be strongly motivated to protect themselves and others from cross-contamination.

Emerging (New) Diseases

A major problem in disease control is the fact that AS ONE DISEASE IS CONTROLLED OR ELIMINATED, SEVERAL NEW ONES ARE DISCOVERED OR OLD ONES EVOLVE TO BECOME SERIOUS. A noted biologist and prize-winning author, Dr. Lewis Thomas, recently wrote:

> There is a lot more research to be done into infectious diseases in general. We have not run out of adversaries, nor is it likely we will do so for a long time to come.

A researcher summarizing problems with AIDS and other diseases stated:

> Microbes, which have existed on this planet for longer than man, show no signs of being unconditionally conquered. Amid the billions that exist harmoniously around us, there will always be some that become unexpectedly disruptive, mysteriously virulent.[1]

Following are examples of recent emerging diseases:

• Acquired Immune Deficiency Syndrome (AIDS)

25

- Creutzfeld Jakob Disease
- Hepatitis B
- Herpes Simplex II
- Legionellosis (Legionnaire's Disease)

These represent the most dangerous category of disease because less may be known about modes of transmission, causative factors and other potential complications than is known about the other categories. The scientific community often has little time to study emerging diseases before public concerns develop. Confusion and fear can distort the facts when the public senses the possibility of an epidemic.

Following are brief descriptions of some emerging diseases and their importance.

Hepatitis Virus B

Hepatitis B, although technically categorized now as an invisible disease, was an emerging disease only a few years ago and is still an excellent example of the latter category.

When the history of infectious diseases important in dentistry is finally written, viral hepatitis B (HBV) may have marked the beginning of a new era in disease challenges to the dental family. Before the advent of HBV, dentistry was primarily concerned with protection of patients from cross-infection from childhood diseases, tuberculosis, influenza, the common cold, syphilis, and gonorrhea. HBV became the catalyst of a new awareness by enlightened dentists and personnel that infectious diseases could be life-threatening to BOTH PATIENTS AND PERSONNEL. Historically, infection control has placed emphasis on preventing the transmission of a disease FROM THE PATIENT TO DENTIST AND/OR STAFF. HBV catalyzed recognition that cross-contamination of everyone involved or associated with dentistry was a realistic possibility.

Although AIDS is presently capturing most of the media headlines and is capturing increasing numbers of infection control research dollars, HBV STILL PRESENTS THE GREATEST THREAT OF ANY PATHOGEN TO DENTISTRY.[2]

A 1983 study of faculty, students, and staff at the University of Colorado School of Dentistry showed that nearly one-third of those tested showed blood "markers."[3] Twenty-nine percent of dentists and staff taking a hepatitis B blood test at the 1983 ADA Annual Meeting showed blood markers.

To a large extent, hepatitis B is largely spread as a population lifestyle disease related, at least in part, to drug and promiscuous sexual activities. Since 1960, the incidence of hepatitis B has become nearly epidemic. In the overall population, five percent of young adults have been exposed, but in large cities the exposure rate may be over twenty percent. In certain foreign countries, the exposure rate among the general population approaches seventy percent.

The incubation period for hepatitis B may be as long as six months or more, and symptoms are absent during this time in more than fifty percent of the cases. Approximately ten percent of the cases become carriers and may remain infective for potentially a lifetime. There are in the United States an estimated two hundred thousand new cases of hepatitis B each year, and there are about a million chronic carriers in the United States. The pool of carriers is continuing to grow from twelve thousand to twenty thousand per year.[4] The seriousness is not limited to the damage done by the disease itself. Studies in India and Africa have shown that the virus remains in the body for years and that this contributes to chronic active hepatitis and cancer of the liver.

A common mode of transmission of hepatitis B is contaminated dental instruments, and a common route of transmission is a cut or a nick on the fingers, through which patients' saliva or blood may infect staff. Blood has been found under the fingernails of treatment personnel for days after completion of treatment. Conversely, dental personnel also may infect patients. Other common modes of transmission include saliva and handpiece spatters and droplets. The virus offers a high risk of cross-contamination because of its high resistance to the environment. *The virus may survive up to a week or longer on contaminated instruments or work surfaces if infection control procedures are inadequate.*[5]

Two vaccines have been developed for hepatitis B which may lead to eradication of the disease. It will be years before the full effect of the vaccines are known. Since the vaccines have proven to be up to ninety percent effective, all health personnel dealing directly with patients should seriously consider vaccination as a preventive measure, if blood testing indicates the need.

The vaccines should be given only in the arm (deltoid muscle), NOT IN THE BUTTOCKS.

Many professionals have been reluctant to be vaccinated for fear of the possibility of acquiring AIDS. The hepatitis B vaccines are made from plasma contributed by chronic carriers, and it is known that one of the highest hepatitis carrier rates is found among male homosexuals—the highest risk group of AIDS.

The risk of acquiring AIDS from the original vaccine is non-existent and has been documented as such by several governmental agencies, including the FDA and the CDC. First, the vaccine is subjected to three different processes to inactivate any known family of viruses which could be present in the plasma from which the vaccine was made. Studies have also shown that HIV, the causative agent of AIDS, does not survive these processes in vaccine production.

Secondly, before the B vaccine was released to the open market, 19,000 individuals were vaccinated in a mass controlled test. Only two individuals developed AIDS, and they were two male homosexuals in New York City. It is probable that these individuals contracted AIDS prior to or subsequent to their receiving the B vaccine.

Furthermore, the higher than average possibility of dental personnel acquiring hepatitis B suggests that treatment personnel, and their immediate family, should give serious consideration to being vaccinated. The Food and Drug Administration certified, in September, 1985, that the vaccine was safe.[6]

In early 1987, an artificially prepared vaccine, Recombivax, became available. Because Recombivax is prepared from "yeast," safety has never been an issue. It is very important that all dental personnel consider being vaccinated with one of the vaccines.

All responsible health organizations, including the Centers for Disease Control (CDC) and the American Dental Association (ADA), have endorsed use of the HBV vaccines by the dental family, and yet the majority of dentists and staff continue to resist vaccination. It is difficult to know if refusal of the vaccines is a result of apathy or a result of a misunderstanding of the risk factors associated with the vaccines. In any event, it is becoming increasingly important that all of the dental family (dentists, hygienists, assistants, students, teachers, lab personnel, supply persons, and family) accept the vaccines. Of course, the major benefit of vaccination is protection from HBV and complications therefrom. However, the hepatitis B virus is being increasingly implicated in other diseases, such as delta hepatitis and more remotely with AIDS.[7]

AS RESEARCH PROGRESSES, THE HBV VACCINES MAY PROVE TO PROVIDE PROTECTION NOT ONLY FROM HBV BUT ALSO FROM SEVERAL RELATED VIRAL DISEASES.

The ADA recently published a compendium of reports on HBV from a symposium held in San Antonio in 1984.[8] The reports contain a substantial amount of information on HBV, and they should be read in their entirety by all dental personnel. Following are a few of the more important excerpts from the publication:

As the prevalence of HBV carriers in the general U.S. population is now 0.7%, an office treating 20 patients per day will encounter one active carrier in every 7 working days.

All persons infected with HBV are potentially infectious to their family, other intimate contacts, and their patients during part of the incubation period and the acute phase of the infection. Infectious potential also exists through the more common subclinical state of the disease when patients are unaware of their infectious status.

Only one in five infected persons has a clinically diagnosed illness. As four of five have had only a subclinical illness, they cannot possibly be aware, or give

27

a history, of hepatitis. Whether they are clinically ill, 10% of infected persons carry the virus for up to a year and 5% remain potentially infectious carriers for several years or the remainder of their lives.

HBV can cause cancer [of the liver].

Infected infants younger than 1 year are much more likely to remain carriers for life. According to Beasley and others, infected children have a 55% risk of death in 30 to 40 years from hepatocellular carcinoma or cirrhosis of the liver. Persistent adult carriers have a 25% rate of death in 20-30 years.

Survival of HBV on a dry surface beyond 7 days demonstrates its ability to remain on operatory clothing worn home and in traces of blood under the fingernails of clinical personnel who do not wear gloves. WITHOUT ADEQUATE PRECAUTIONS, IT MAY BE POSSIBLE FOR EVEN IMMUNIZED OPERATORY PERSONNEL TO TRANSMIT DURABLE INFECTIOUS AGENTS SUCH AS HBV TO FAMILY OR OTHER INTIMATE CONTACTS.

And from a dental hygienist who became a carrier:

In the matter of 2 short months, my entire life changed. Suddenly, I was completely unemployed with no means of support. When you're educated to be a dental hygienist, that is all you're trained to do. I lost a sense of being a useful, contributing human being. I was suddenly at home every day with nothing to do, just a lot of time on my hands, and wondering what I would do for the rest of my life. This led to a period of deep depression.

I have had 2 years now to adjust to the fact that I am a carrier and, most likely, will always be a carrier because I have retained the surface antigen

now for 2 years and am e antigen positive. But some of the factors are still difficult for me to accept. Knowing my chances of liver disease are highly increased is hard to deal with, along with feelings of being a potential threat to friends and family and having to be constantly "on guard" when visiting in people's homes or playing with their children.

My point is extremely simple. The risks that you run are not worth the consequences you may have to face.

And from a dentist who became an HBV carrier:

My exposure [to HBV] occurred sometime between spring and early summer 1981. My contact was, I believe, the result of failure to use common sense and to follow routine preventive procedures.

The personal effects of hepatitis are, to me, noticeable and devastating. I wish I could find the words to express clearly to you what it is like, physically and emotionally, to daily find yourself exhausted. My energy level has failed me. It is difficult to last a full day at work. Usually by 2:00 p.m. I feel like someone has pulled a plug and I can feel the energy drain from me like water from a tub.

Physically, I am more susceptible to a variety of illnesses; my body's resistance is compromised. I am limited to a narrower choice of medications when needed because of the negative effect many drugs have on the liver. I live with the knowledge that I am more than 275 times more likely to develop hepatocellular carcinoma than the average person.

These problems and the negative effects they can have on your life and the lives of your family are avoidable. The choice is up to you. You are fortunate that you still have a choice.

As illustrated by the excerpts from the personal experiences quoted above, *THE EFFECTS OF*

HBV (AND OTHER SIMILAR DISEASES) CAN BE WIDESPREAD, INCLUDING INTERRUPTION OF INCOME, PSYCHOLOGICAL DEVASTATION, INVOLVEMENT OF LOVED ONES, DETERIORATING HEALTH, AND DEATH. The dental family must observe all infection control precautions possible, including vaccination and implementation of an efficacious program of precautionary procedures to prevent such critical problems.

Herpes Simplex I and II (Genital)

As with viral hepatitis, herpes virus infections have evolved from mere inconveniences to increasing degrees of seriousness. Historically, herpes had meant primarily the presence of cold sores to dentistry. In the past several decades, herpes has evolved, perhaps through mutation, to a number of very serious threats to dentistry, including the following:

Herpetic Whitlow

Herpetic Whitlow is a form of herpes simplex I or herpes simplex II which infects the fingers and results in the loss of countless man-hours of productive dental office time each year and in excruciating pain for those infected.

Herpetic Whitlow is often considered primarily an infection of the fingers of dentists or dental auxiliaries. Actually, other professions have a problem of comparable severity. The January, 1984, *American Journal of Nursing* (Lucey, pp. 60-61) reported on three cases of Whitlow infection in nurses. Etiologies were a blister from guitar playing and paper cuts, which became infected and resulted in incapacitation of one nurse for two and one-half weeks, one for three and one-half weeks and one for four weeks. In two cases, tenderness of the infected finger persisted for five months and, in one case, tenderness was still present after eighteen months.

The incubation period of Herpetic Whitlow is two to twelve days. The infection is first manifested by a tingling in the involved finger, followed by intense, constant throbbing pain that is extremely severe. The area is red and swollen and the pulp space is soft, not tense. Vesicles erupt and may ulcerate or coalesce, and new satellite vesicles may appear. The clear, infectious fluid in the vesicles may change to cloudy, but it is not purulent. Fever, chills and malaise may precede the infection's onset or may accompany the acute phase. Lymphadenopathy and lymphangitis may be present, the latter denoted by a red streak that travels up the hand into the forearm.

Because Whitlow is rare, except in certain populations such as dentistry, the infection is often misdiagnosed. It is advisable to suggest the possibility of Whitlow to physicians treating dental personnel for finger infections.

HERPETIC WHITLOW IS AN OCCUPATIONAL HAZARD OF DENTISTRY WHICH CAN BE PRACTICALLY ERADICATED WITH GLOVING. AT THE VERY LEAST, PERSONNEL WITH CUTS, NICKS OR ABRASIONS OF THE FINGERS SHOULD COVER THE INJURIES WITH LATEX FINGERCOTS UNTIL HEALED.

Herpetic Conjunctivitis

Herpes of the eye is another variation of herpes I or II which is potentially very serious to dentistry. The herpes virus being splashed into the eye during a drilling, grinding, or polishing procedure, or the herpes virus being wiped into the eye from contaminated fingers of staff rubbing their eyes during treatment, can result in blindness of the infected eye.

As evidenced by the "If Saliva Were Red," previously described in Chapter 2, dental procedures often contaminate much of the treatment area with splashes, aerosols, wipes, and touches leaving blood, serum, saliva, and other debris on surfaces and equipment. Heads of treatment personnel are always within the range of the "septic spray," and, as a result, eyes of dentists and treatment staff are always susceptible to infection from flying pathogens.

IT IS VERY IMPORTANT THAT DENTAL TREATMENT PERSONNEL WEAR EYE PROTECTION DURING TREATMENT PROCEDURES AND THAT PERSONNEL

DO NOT TOUCH OR WIPE EYES UNTIL HANDS HAVE BEEN WASHED AFTER TREATMENT WITH AN ANTIMICROBIAL SOAP.

Herpetic Cold Sores

Dentistry has historically considered cold sores as occasional, unavoidable herpes aggravations. However, it is possible for even the usually less serious forms of herpes to result in serious consequences. A study was reported in the *Journal of the American Medical Association*[9] detailing a case of a dental hygienist who transmitted herpes simplex I to more than 20 patients. This is the first study confirming that a form of herpes can cross-infect humans in the dental office.

The hygienist causing the cross-infection had contracted the herpes through a chronic skin rash, and she had then treated patients without using gloves as a barrier between herself and the patients. The result was the infection of 20 patients over a four-day period. Many of the patients who became infected developed a prolonged fever, severe sore throat and weight loss.

Previous research has shown that medical and dental personnel are at increased risk of contracting herpes. While it has not been demonstrated that herpes II is transmitted through blood, saliva, and body fluids in the dental office, there are many similarities between herpes II, herpes I, and other viral diseases, for example hepatitis B. Dental personnel must assume that all herpes infections MAY be dentally transmitted, and treatment of patients with visible lesions should be delayed whenever possible.[10]

A vaccine for simplex I has been tested successfully in laboratory mice, and research conducted at the National Institutes of Health has shown that this genetically engineered vaccine may prevent development of a latent infection.[11] Although the vaccine is directed against simplex I, it appears to also provide protection against simplex II (venereal herpes).

The October 13, 1984, issue of the *Canada Diseases Weekly Report* compared cases of herpes in Canada in 1983 to similar reporting periods beginning with 1978. The comparisons are quite revealing in that the 10,237 reported cases of all types of herpes was an increase of nearly 700 percent from 1978 and 64 percent from 1982. Possible reasons for the increases were listed as follows:

1. Increased medical consultation by symptomatic persons.

2. Increased demand by the medical profession for laboratory confirmation of infection.

3. Prenatal screening as a preventive measure for neo-natal herpes.

4. Increased frequency of genital herpes virus infection.

The probability is that the increase reflects a combination of the four cited possibilities.

The greatest increase was in children under six months of age (143 percent) with a fatality rate of 9.1 percent. Neo-natal herpes is a very serious complication of herpes II (venereal herpes). Infection of newborn can be partially controlled by caesarian birth, but a large percentage of children born accordingly still contract the disease.

The Canadian studies also showed that females are more susceptible to contracting herpes. The increase in female cases from 1982 to 1983 was 81 percent and in male cases 57 percent. The female-male ratio by age was:

Age	Ratio
15-19	13:1
20-24	3:1
25-29	1.5:1

Canada's experience is similar to that of other advanced countries of the world. Herpes must be dealt with as a truly threatening disease, and dentistry is a high risk group for contracting and transmitting herpes. It has been shown that the herpes virus is transmitted in all body fluids and that it is highly contagious under certain circumstances. Herpes viruses has also been shown to survive from hours to days in the dental environment.

STERILIZATION, SURFACE DISINFECTION AND GLOVING ARE THREE INDISPENSIBLE PRECAUTIONS WHICH HELP PREVENT THE DENTAL TRANSMISSION OF HERPES.

Herpes Simplex II (Genital Herpes)

Herpes simplex II is an emerging disease which has had great impact on human lifestyle. Data from the Centers for Disease Control showed a ninety percent increase in visits of herpes patients to private physicians in 1983. Growth is slowing but is still substantial. It is estimated that there are approximately 20,000,000 cases of herpes II in the United States alone.[12] Primarily considered a venereal disease, herpes II can be devastating to the victims who suffer periodic outbreaks as often as five to eight times a year, with each occurrence lasting about three weeks. Symptoms include ulcerated lesions, extreme pain, fever, genital discharge, and general malaise. Lesions occur on the genital area, buttocks, fingers, thighs, and occasionally on other parts of the body. There is some indication that herpes II may be predisposing to cancer of the female cervix.[13]

The disease may lie dormant for years, and it is often passed from infected mothers to their newborn. Approximately fifty percent of the babies of mothers infected with herpes II are born with the disease, and about twenty-five percent of such newborns develop severe complications, such as mental retardation or death.[14]

Little is known about many aspects of herpes simplex II, and there is no cure available, although some researchers have reported progress on a vaccine. A new drug, generically named acyclovir with the brand name Zovirax, by Burroughs-Wellcome, is helpful in reducing the symptoms of herpes II. If administered when symptoms first appear and before vesicles mature, duration of the herpes II outbreak is shortened by approximately 50%. Effectiveness reduces with multiple treatment.

Some dental practitioners are experimenting with acyclovir in the treatment of herpes simplex I with some apparent success in reducing the severity of cold sores. However, the herpes virus has been shown to mutate relatively easily and is resistant to newer forms of therapy. As such, some experts are currently recommending that Zovirax (generically acyclovir) be reserved only for those herpes cases which are severe or life-threatening. Other modes of therapy, such as L-Lysine, although somewhat less effective, should be used for localized, recurrent episodes.

Studies show that modes of transmission of herpes may be more diverse than originally thought. There is also some evidence that herpes may be transmitted through various body fluids, possibly in the same ways as hepatitis. For example, herpes II virus has now been shown to be present in saliva, even when no lesions are present in the mouth. Dental personnel may have greater exposure to herpes simplex II than originally thought, and they must be wary of potential problems.

Cytomegalovirus

Cytomegalovirus (CMV) is a member of the broad family of herpes or herpes-like viruses and is the causative agent of several infectious disease problems potentially related to practitioners and staff. CMV has also been identified as a source of major infection of the unborn and newborn infants.

According to the federal Centers for Disease Control in Atlanta, cytomegalovirus is the most common type of prenatal infection. It is the leading known cause of congenital hearing problems, and a major cause of mental retardation.

Approximately 90 percent of the time, CMV is harmless to healthy children and adults, who may show no symptoms or only cold-like symptoms. Most of the time a fetus will also escape unscathed, but in about one in ten cases, the virus attacks the central nervous system of the unborn child. One study estimated that 7,000 American newborns each year suffer neurological disorders attributable to CMV infections contracted in the womb.

CMV is also a threat to people whose immune systems are suppressed, including premature newborns and organ and bone marrow transplant recipients receiving immunosuppressant drugs to prevent rejection of the transplant. In them, the virus can trigger severe lung and liver infections, including hepatitis and pneumonia. As the use of immunosuppressive drugs continues to grow, as in the treatment of diabetes and with transplantation of organs, CMV may continue to spread in adults.

CMV is not a new disease, but the conditions under which it spreads most rapidly are. As increasing numbers of pre-toilet trained children are grouped in close contact with one another in day care centers, CMV is spreading rapidly among these toddlers who can spread it through urine, feces or saliva to the young women who typically care for them, many of whom may be planning families.

An estimated seven million American children between ages three and five attend day care centers, sharing diapering and meal facilities and toys. Massachusetts alone has about 1,100 day care centers and 9,000 day care homes, according to Katherine Messenger, unit director of the Massachusetts Preschool and School Health Service.

A dramatic disparity between CMV infection rates among children at day care centers and those cared for at home has been shown in recent studies. In one 1984 study in Alabama, only 18 percent of the children at home showed evidence of the virus, compared to 57 percent at a wealthy suburban day care center. A single child can continue to shed the virus and infect others for months or sometimes years.

"The results suggested that almost all of the children in this setting would acquire the virus," concluded Dr. Robert Pass, a University of Alabama pediatrician whose studies on CMV have been published in the *New England Journal of Medicine, Pediatrics* and other journals.

The incidence of CMV has been rising since it first was isolated in the 1950s, but trends now indicate that a generation from now, nearly all Americans will have been exposed to CMV as children, acquiring permanent immunity. "This is a one-point-in-time phenomenon," Messenger said.

But for young women today who chose careers working with very young children, as may be the case in dentistry—particularly in pedo and ortho—fear of contracting CMV may prompt some dental staff to quit work if they are hoping to become pregnant. *Such action is not necessary if basic infection control procedures are practiced.* Medical literature cites at least two healthcare workers who opted for abortions after contracting the disease from nursery children during pregnancy.

Not only day care workers are at risk. The May 29, 1986 issue of the *New England Journal of Medicine* stated: "Children often transmit CMV to parents and could be an important source of maternal CMV infection during pregnancy."

Because of the increasing popularity of day care centers, "infants and preschoolers are now acquiring infections at an earlier age than previously," a 1984 report in the *Journal of the American Medical Association* said. As well as colds, flu and CMV, hepatitis and diarrheal disease are easily spread among toddlers at day care centers.

Like the other herpes viruses, such as those that cause chicken pox and cold sores, CMV may become latent, remaining inactive in the cells it infects and possibly re-erupting later, with uncertain consequences.

The greatest unknown, however, is CMV's effect on the individual developing fetus. Its invisible and endemic nature makes it hard to track. Because a woman is unlikely to know she has the disease while pregnant, notes Robert Matousek, March of Dimes Birth Defects Foundations statistician, any disorders in her child may be impossible to trace to CMV. *The cause of 60 percent of all birth defects is unknown.*

Several institutions have been trying to develop a vaccine against CMV, with little success. Herpes viruses are a unique problem in terms of immunization, researchers say, partly because of the latency. The herpes virus that causes chicken pox, for example, can re-erupt in old age as shingles.

Immune globulin promises the best short-term protection against CMV. Supported in part by a grant from the National Institutes of Health, the blood product has been undergoing human trials for more than three years at seven hospitals. More than 30 kidney transplant patients have shown no adverse side-effects since they were treated with the globulin.

Dental personnel, particularly women, should exercise careful infection control procedures when working on younger children who are cared for in day care centers or who have contact with larger groups of other children where body fluids may be exchanged. In addition to office personnel, others at risk of possible exposure to CMV, and other organisms, are laboratory personnel who handle contaminated impressions, models, and other materials transmitted from dental offices not disinfecting such items. All incoming devices, models, impressions and other items which have been removed from the oral cavity should be disinfected before being handled by laboratory personnel. CMV is also a potential threat to such personnel, partly because the virus has been shown to survive for days on dried surfaces.

Tuberculosis

Tuberculosis continues to be an increasing concern in the United States. As previously noted, most health agencies reported years ago that TB would continue to decline and would no longer be a major health threat in the U.S. by approximately the year 2010. A few years ago, the decrease in new cases of tuberculosis began to level off. So far in 1986, new cases of tuberculosis exceed last year by approximately 500 cases. Five hundred new cases of TB may not seem significant; however, if these 500 cases are added to the previously projected decline in cases, *the increase is very significant.*

Table 3 illustrates the turn-around in tuberculosis. It should be noted that new cases exceed the projected cases in every category, ranging from an increase over projection of from 3.6%-25.7%. This overall increase illustrates that the problem is not isolated but

exists generally throughout the population of the United States.

Tuberculosis has been identified by a study reported in a July, 1986 *New England Journal of Medicine* as a possible prodromal symptom of AIDS. The authors stated that TB can appear up to five years ahead of other symptoms in persons infected with HIV.

Additionally, the Centers for Disease Control recently reported that preliminary data indicates that approximately ten percent of AIDS patients may have tuberculosis. Dr. Dixie Snider, Jr., head of the CDC's TB control division, stated, "We are seeing more TB in areas with the most AIDS cases, and it's now firmly established that a form of TB does strike AIDS patients."

One theory by researchers in Florida is that the suppressed immune system of AIDS patients allows the reactivation of formerly dormant tubercular lesions. Because TB may prove to be an AIDS "tag-along" infection, dentistry must be particularly aware of identifying the disease. Dentistry has been shown to be a primary discipline for possibly identifying AIDS patients because of the high incidence of early intra-oral manifestations of the disease.

Table 4 compares actual to predicted cases of tuberculosis from 1982 to June 15, 1986.

Acquired Immunodeficiency Syndrome (AIDS)

Acquired immunodeficiency syndrome (AIDS) is the latest and the most deadly of the emerging diseases. The startling speed with which the disease has developed has led some researchers to compare the spread of AIDS to the spread of plagues in the Middle Ages. At the least, AIDS has the potential of being the most serious infectious disease of modern times. The public awareness of AIDS has progressed with startling speed. It is nearly impossible to read a newspaper or a magazine, to listen to the radio, or to watch television without seeing or hearing a reference to AIDS.

Public awareness of AIDS seems to have begun

TABLE 3
Comparison of Observed (Reported) and Expected Tuberculosis Cases by Age Group, Sex, Race, and Ethnicity
United States, 1985 vs. 1984

	Observed Cases 1984	Observed Cases 1985	Expected Cases 1985	Observed More Than Expected	Percent
Age					
◀5..............	759	789	700	+ 89	+ 12.7
5-14..............	477	472	417	+ 55	+ 13.2
15-24..............	1,682	1,672	1,526	+ 146	+ 9.6
25-44..............	6,409	6,764	6,101	+ 663	+ 10.9
45-64	6,427	6,143	5,932	+ 211	+ 3.6
65 + ...	6,501	6,361	6,117	+ 244	+ 4.0
Sex					
Male..............	14,441	14,499	13,488	+ 1,011	+ 7.5
Female.............	7,814	7,702	7,283	+ 419	+ 5.8
Race					
White..............	11,729	11,538	10,791	+ 747	+ 6.9
Black..............	7,678	7,734	7,440	+ 294	+ 4.0
Asian/Pacific Islander	2,473	2,532	2,238	+ 294	+ 13.1
American Indian/Alaskan					
Native.............	375	397	339	+ 58	+ 17.1
Ethnicity					
Hispanic	2,750	3,134	2,494	+ 640	+ 25.7
Non-Hispanic	19,505	19,067	18,276	+ 791	+ 4.3

Courtesy Centers for Disease Control

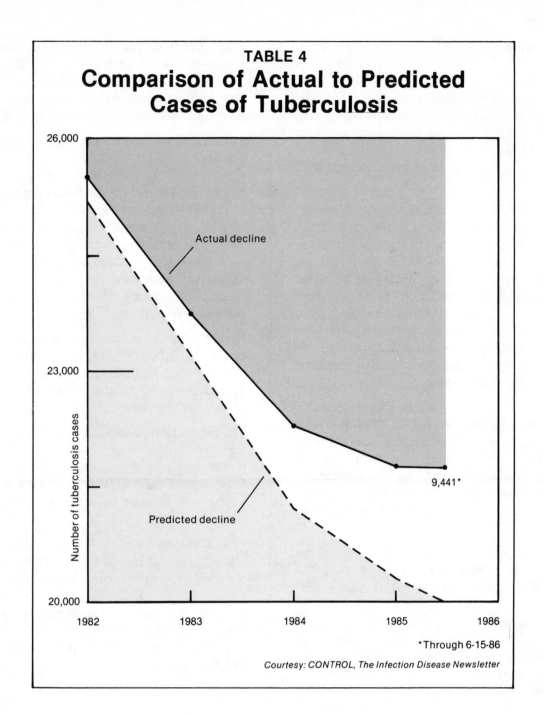

TABLE 4
Comparison of Actual to Predicted Cases of Tuberculosis

Number of tuberculosis cases

Actual decline

Predicted decline

9,441*

26,000

23,000

20,000

1982   1983   1984   1985   1986

*Through 6-15-86

Courtesy: CONTROL, The Infection Disease Newsletter

35

with a statement in 1983 that "the U.S. Government's top health official said today that AIDS has become the number one priority of the United States Public Health Service."[15] Public awareness escalated since that time until the disclosure in June, 1985, and subsequent death in October, 1985, of Mr. Rock Hudson, a world renowned actor, that he was afflicted with AIDS.

Following the announcement by Mr. Hudson, the public media were flooded with stories on AIDS, some accurate and some misleading, emphasizing the potential effect of AIDS on various segments of society. What may be called the "Hudson Syndrome" may prove to have catalyzed interest and additional research into the deadly disease. Pressure from the public for a cure has already attracted additional research dollars that were being more slowly released until the Hudson Syndrome.

For the first time ever, an infectious disease, AIDS, was the subject of a Gallup Poll[16] reporting that 95% of the persons polled across the United States had heard of AIDS, an increase of 18% in two years. Very significantly, 66% of the persons polled reported that they "expected AIDS to spread to all kinds of people in our country."

If public pressure of AIDS continues at the present level, many side benefits may be realized. Because the disease is correctly perceived as primarily a venereal, drug-abuse, homosexual, blood-transferred disease, fear of contracting the disease may have a beneficial effect on certain segments of society. There is already evidence that sexual promiscuity on some college campuses is lessening as a result of the AIDS scare. It is possible that one side benefit to publicity of AIDS will be a substantial reduction of sexually transmitted diseases (STD).

Spread of AIDS

AIDS is developing in almost epidemic proportions. From January, 1979, to April 16, 1984, 4087 cases of AIDS were reported in the U.S. and Puerto Rico. From April 16, 1984, to August 2, 1985, cases increased to nearly 12,000. Almost one-third of all cases of AIDS identified were reported in the first half of 1985. And AIDS cases doubled in the first half of 1985 as compared to the same reporting period in 1984.

Perhaps even more serious, researchers are predicting that AIDS cases will continue to double yearly or more often for at least the next few years. Table 5 on the following page graphically illustrates growth of the disease, by quarter, since identification of the disease in 1979. The almost geometric growth is evident in such illustration. Fortunately, most recent data suggests that growth in the blood transfuse-related and perhaps homosexual populations are beginning to plateau.

Researchers continue to estimate that an estimated 2,000,000 or more Americans are infected with HIV, the causative agent of AIDS and that over 50 percent of persons in the ARC Stage II of the disease will eventually die.

The incubation period of AIDS has continued to increase until it is now speculated that incubation may be up to a lifetime and that persons may carry HIV for a month, a year, ten years, or a lifetime before moving through the stages to death.

Dramatic growth of AIDS is not limited to the United States. Most of Europe has shown a percentage growth of the disease equal to the United States as illustrated by Table 6. Additionally, the disease has continued to spread around the world, with over 130 World Health Organization nations reporting presence of the disease.

Evolution of AIDS

AIDS has been found predominantly in high risk groups, particularly sexually promiscuous male homosexuals, drug-abusers, other sexually promiscuous persons, and individuals who require multiple blood transfusions. However, research in Africa suggests that the disease may also be transmitted by sexual and non-sexual family contact. Of the 124 cases of AIDS studied in Africa to date, 110 or 89% have no known

TABLE 5
AIDS Cases By Quarter — United States

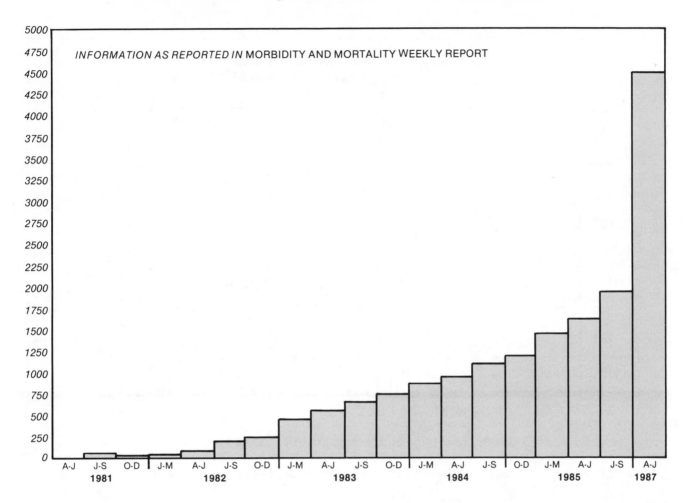

INFORMATION AS REPORTED IN MORBIDITY AND MORTALITY WEEKLY REPORT

risk factor. This suggestion of transmission by family or other close contact is potentially more serious because it is believed that AIDS may have originated in Africa. AIDS in Africa may have had more time to mature to a disease of normal lifestyles. If so, the possibility exists that the U.S. may also experience an evolution of AIDS into normal lifestyle populations. Present evidence in the U.S. does not suggest transmission by casual contact.

It is speculated that AIDS originated in Africa as a result of a monkey infecting a human, thereby transmitting Simian AIDS to the human. Presumably, migration of the disease to the U.S. occurred when homosexual contacts in Africa traveled through Haiti and then infected homosexual partners in the United States. If this

scenario and evolution prove to be correct, the information may be important because researchers may utilize such data to accelerate development of a vaccine or other cure.

Stages of AIDS

The incubation period of AIDS varies and has been shown to be potentially a lifetime.[17] The wide range of incubation periods helps explain the perceived discrepancies in the confirmed number of approximate 40,000 cases of "Classical" AIDS and the estimated 2,000,000 + or more persons infected with the HIV virus. Many persons carrying the virus will not know that they are infected until the appearance of symp-

TABLE 6
AIDS Cases and Number of Deaths

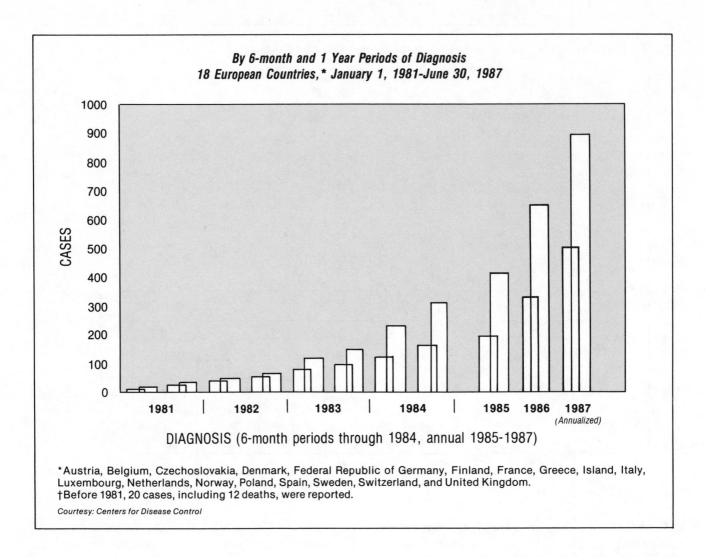

By 6-month and 1 Year Periods of Diagnosis
18 European Countries,* January 1, 1981-June 30, 1987

DIAGNOSIS (6-month periods through 1984, annual 1985-1987)

*Austria, Belgium, Czechoslovakia, Denmark, Federal Republic of Germany, Finland, France, Greece, Island, Italy, Luxembourg, Netherlands, Norway, Poland, Spain, Sweden, Switzerland, and United Kingdom.
†Before 1981, 20 cases, including 12 deaths, were reported.

Courtesy: Centers for Disease Control

toms encourages them to seek diagnosis in future years.

As a result of the high level of public interest in AIDS, much misinformation is being disseminated. It is important to clearly understand the facts concerning AIDS, as presently perceived. Without accurate information, dental personnel cannot make a considered decision as to whether they will treat AIDS or AIDS-related patients in the various stages of the disease.

Scientific evidence[18] presently suggests at least three stages of the disease (summarized in Table 7 on the following page):

1. STAGE ONE occurs when a person becomes infected with the HIV virus and the person appears to live compatibly with the virus. Few, if any, symptoms are exhibited during Stage 1, and infected persons live a relatively uncomplicated life, except for the possible psychological trauma of not knowing if the infection may evolve into the other two stages.

It has not been confirmed if persons in Stage 1 are able to infect others, but the evidence suggests that anyone infected with the virus, in any stage, may infect others. There is also a suggestion in some studies that persons in Stage 1 may be the most infectious because of a higher titer of the virus in body fluids.

TABLE 7
Stages and Symptoms of AIDS

STAGE 1 — VIRUS RELATED

1. Should not be called AIDS. This Stage is really "Virus-related" with few if any symptoms.
2. Patients live uncomplated lives but may be infectious to others.
3. May cause extreme mental trauma because those infected do not now when or if the disease will progress to other Stages.

STAGE 2 — AIDS RELATED COMPLEX (ARC)

1. General malaise.
2. Mild weight loss.
3. Occasional fever.
4. Occasional cough.
5. Some skin infections.
6. Slightly swollen lymph nodes (primarily neck).
7. Shingles.
8. Intra-oral hairy leukoplakia.
9. Lowered resistance to infections.

STAGE 3 — CLASSIC AIDS

1. General malaise.
2. Persistent diarrhea.
3. Persistent chronic cough.
4. Persistent fever.
5. Night sweats and insomnia.
6. Burning during urination.
7. Progressive weakness.
8. Occasional persistent purplish rash or bruises on body.
9. Leukopenia.
10. Shingles.
11. Swollen lymph nodes (particularly neck).
12. Intra-oral manifestations:
    a. Hairy leukoplakia.
    b. Candidiasis.
    c. Legionella.
    d. Herpes simplex I.
    e. Kaposi's sarcoma.
    f. Squamous cell carcinoma.
    g. Oral lesions of other venereal diseases.
    h. Sputums are usually positive for pneumocystis carinii.

Certain oral symptoms, discussed more fully later in this chapter, may predict infection with the virus. Preliminary data suggests that over 50 percent of persons in Stage 1 may progress to Stage 2 (ARC) or Stage 3 (Classical AIDS).

2. STAGE TWO, called AIDS-related complex (ARC), occurs when persons are infected with HIV but present a milder version of the disease, with less severe symptoms than those of Classical AIDS.

Symptoms of Stage 2 ARC include a mild version of the immune-system depression with a lowered resistance to various infections. Those infected begin to miss work. Additionally, infected persons show general malaise, mild weight loss, occasional fever, mild cough, skin infections, shingles, hairy leukoplakia, and swollen lymph nodes. Such symptoms may be confused with other illnesses.

Persons with ARC may remain in Stage 2 of the disease apparently indefinitely, or they may progress to Stage 3. Researchers are studying why certain infected persons remain in Stage 2 and certain others evolve into Stage 3. Some investigators theorize that ADDITIONAL VIRAL OR MICROBIAL INFECTIONS MAY PLAY A ROLE IN THE PROGRESSION OF AIDS. Suspected contributors, triggers, or co-agents include Epstein-Barr virus and cytomegalovirus (both members of the herpes family), and the hepatitis B virus.[19]

It is very questionable as to whether the hepatitis B virus may be involved as a co-agent with AIDS. However, if such is the case, DENTAL PERSONNEL WHO ACCEPT THE HEPATITIS B VACCINE MAY BE AFFORDED PROTECTION FROM STAGE 3 AIDS if they later become infected with HIV. One of the AIDS research challenges is to determine whether other viruses are co-agents activating AIDS or whether the other viruses are present because of infections encouraged by the lowered immunity resulting from the presence of the HIV virus.

Present data suggests that up to 100 percent of persons in Stage 2 ARC will progress to Stage 3 Classical AIDS.

3. STAGE THREE is the Classical, full infection of AIDS with symptoms of fever, night sweats, loss of weight, diarrhea, uncomfortable urination, persistent cough, general malaise, progressive weakness, leukopenia, an occasional purplish skin rash somewhat resembling a bruise or group of bruises, shingles, swollen lymph nodes, hairy leukoplakia, and other oral symptoms as discussed on the following pages.

It is estimated that ALL persons in Stage 3 AIDS will die. Although only approximately 50 percent of those persons reported to have had AIDS to date are dead, over 80 percent of the persons diagnosed before 1983 have died.[20] The projected high mortality rate suggests that ALL individuals with Second Stage ARC may progress to Stage Three AIDS. Until a more meaningful statistical base is available, mortality projections will remain speculative. However, there is no doubt that *AIDS is the most deadly disease ever to confront dentistry.*

Because a lack of understanding of AIDS may result in a purely emotional view of the disease, it is very important that dental personnel fully understand the stages of AIDS. VARYING LEVELS OF RISK MAY EXIST WITH PERSONS INFECTED WITH THE HIV AIDS VIRUS. ACCORDINGLY, DENTAL PERSONNEL MAY WISH TO CONSIDER WHETHER THEY WILL TREAT STAGE 3 AIDS PATIENTS, STAGE 2 ARC PATIENTS, STAGE 1 HIV INFECTED PATIENTS, OR NO AIDS-RELATED PATIENTS. Such choices may not be necessary at the present time, but the probability is that dentistry will be faced with such choices in the near future as more infected persons are identified. Increasing numbers of infected persons, possibly in the millions, may force such choices.

Oral Symptoms of AIDS

Dentistry may be on the front line in the diagnosis of Stage 2 or Stage 3 AIDS. The Centers for Disease Control reported[21] that:

> *Hairy leukoplakia may be of diagnostic value as an early indicator of HIV infections, especially when*

observed in combination with other clinical findings. APPROXIMATELY 95% OF PATIENTS WITH AIDS (STAGE 3) OR ARC (STAGE 2) ARE REPORTED TO HAVE CERVICAL LYMPHADENOPATHY AND OTHER HEAD AND NECK MANIFESTATIONS OF THE DISEASE, WHICH MAY BE DETECTED BY DENTISTS AND OTHERS UNDERTAKING ORAL OR FACIAL EXAMINATION.

Health-care providers, INCLUDING DENTAL PERSONNEL, are in a unique position to identify clinical oral symptoms and their potential association with AIDS.

AIDS patients die primarily from opportunistic infections overcoming the weakened immune system of the body. Oral symptoms include oral candidiasis, hairy leukoplakia, oral herpes simplex, oral legionella, oral lesions from syphilis and gonorrhea, Kaposi's sarcoma, squamous cell carcinoma, and lymphoma. Although not a true oral manifestation, sputum cultures are usually positive for *Pneumocystis carinii* early in Stage 1 or Stage 2 of AIDS.

Hairy leukoplakia, a relatively rare oral condition, has been detected in a number of AIDS patients and may be an early indicator of the disease.[22] The condition appears as raised white areas on the lateral border of the tongue. Seventy-eight of 79 persons tested with hairy leukoplakia at a San Francisco health center showed signs of having been exposed to HIV, and at least 42 of a group of 123 patients with the condition actually developed AIDS.[23] Candida has been reported on the surface of the leukoplakia lesions, as have a number of other viruses including papilloma, herpes, and Epstein-Barr.

Oral findings are important early diagnostic tools for dentists and other healthcare providers in the identification and treatment of AIDS.

As evidenced by the data above, studies are showing a very high incidence of oral manifestations early in the diagnosis of AIDS. In addition to the fact that 95% of all AIDS patients show symptoms in the head or neck, preliminary evidence suggests that over 50% of Stage 3 AIDS patients may seek diagnosis because of intra-oral symptoms. If such preliminary data is confirmed, DENTISTRY MAY WELL BE ON THE FRONT-LINE OF POSSIBLE EXPOSURE TO THE HIV VIRUS THROUGH NOT ONLY DENTAL TREATMENT (PRIMARILY INVOLVING BLOOD), BUT ALSO THROUGH EXPOSURE TO GROWING NUMBERS OF DISGUISED AND UNDIAGNOSED AIDS PATIENTS SEEKING DIAGNOSIS OF ORAL SYMPTOMS OF THE DISEASE. Even though probability of either exposure may be minimal at the present time, it is prudent for dental personnel to recognize that the possibility exists and that the possibility will increase in the next several years.

Transmission and Dentistry

On June 4, 1987, a physician announced at the Third International Conference on AIDS, Washington, D.C., that a dentist had contracted AIDS as a result of dental practice. At this writing, scientific details are still forthcoming; however, the announcement stated that the dentist was not subject to other high risk modes of transmission and that the dentist had contracted the HIV infection from treating an HIV patient(s) in his dental practice. The announcement further stated that the disease was probably contracted *"through cuts on the hands and fingers"* because the dentist did not wear gloves.

This announcement that a dentist had contracted AIDS from dental practice was released only 13 days after publication of the report by the Centers for Disease Control (CDC) concerning the three most recent healthcare workers who were infected by HIV without high risk exposure. Following are excerpts from the CDC report:[24]

> WORKER 1: A female healthcare worker assisting with an unsuccessful attempt to insert an arterial catheter in a patient suffering a cardiac arrest . . . applied pressure to the insertion site to

stop the bleeding. During the procedure, she may have had a small amount of blood on her index finger for about 20 minutes before washing her hands. Afterwards, she may also have assisted in cleaning the room but did not recall any other exposures to the patient's blood or body fluids. She had no open wounds, but her hands were chapped. Although she often wore gloves when anticipating exposure to blood, she was not wearing gloves during this incident.

A postmortem examination [of the patient] . . . was positive for HIV antibody. Twenty days after the incident, the healthcare worker became ill. The illness lasted three weeks. She had donated blood six months before the incident and was negative for HIV. She donated again 16 weeks after the incident and was positive for HIV.

WORKER 2: A female phlebotomist was filling a 10 ml vacuum blood collection tube with blood from an outpatient with suspected HIV infection when the top of the tube flew off and blood splattered around the room, on her face, and in her mouth. She was wearing gloves . . . and was wearing eyeglasses so she did not think she got blood in her eyes. She washed the blood off immediately after exposure. The outpatient's blood sample was positive for HIV antibody. The phlebotomist was negative [for HIV] the day after the incident and again eight weeks later. When she donated blood nine months later, she was positive.

WORKER 3: A female medical technologist was manipulating a blood-component separating machine . . . when blood spilled, covering most of her hands and forearms. She was not wearing gloves. She does not recall having open wounds on her hands or [having] any mucous membrane exposure. However, she

had dermatitis on one ear and may have touched it. . .a blood sample from the patient was positive for HIV antibody. The technologist's tests were negative five days after exposure and again six weeks later. Eight weeks after exposure, she had an influenza-like illness . . . which resolved after a few weeks. Three months after the incident, she was positive for HIV antibody.

The editor's note appended to the above report prepared by the CDC Hospital Infections Program and AIDS Program stated:

Three instances of healthcare workers with HIV infections associated with skin or mucous-membrane exposure to blood from HIV-infected patients are reported above. Careful investigation of these three cases is not known . . . The three cases reported here suggest that exposure of skin or mucous membranes to contaminated blood may rarely result in transmission of HIV. *The magnitude of risk is not known . . . the increasing prevalence of HIV infection increases the potential for such exposures, especially when routinely recommended precautions are not followed.*

These four new cases (if the HIV-dentist infection case withstands investigation) of non-high risk transmission of HIV to healthcare workers, coupled with the previously CDC reported six healthcare worker transmission cases, emphasize the need for *all* healthcare workers, *including those associated with dentistry,* to intensify their infection control procedures. The ten investigated cases all had several commonalities:

1. Each person was exposed by blood contact, either through needle puncture, through a skin rash (or dermatitis), or through a mucous membrane.

2. Each person was exposed by *direct contact*. To date, no cases of HIV transmission have been recorded where personnel utilized efficacious barrier techniques, including gloving, masking, and wearing eye protection.

These four cases are significant to dentistry. Several facts and reasonable assumptions should be noted:

1. HIV transmission apparently requires the presence of blood products, and, because dental treatment personnel routinely work in the presence of blood, theoretical exposure to HIV must be considered. *Wearing barrier gloves during treatment minimizes or eliminates such risk.*

2. Because one of the four healthcare workers was apparently contaminated by blood through the mucous membrane, it must be considered that cross-contamination from HIV-infected dental personnel working intraorally is at least a remote possibility. *Wearing barrier gloves and masks during treatment minimizes or eliminates such risk.* Had the infected healthcare worker worn a mask, the possibility of infection through her mouth would have been minimized or eliminated.

3. It is significant that the CDC editor stated: *The magnitude of risk is not known . . . the increasing prevalence of HIV infection increases the potential for such exposures, especially when routinely recommended precautions are not followed.* The obvious intent of such a statement is to emphasize that much is still to be learned about HIV transmission and that it is very important to practice disciplined infection control procedures when treating AIDS patients.

Dentistry should maintain a reasonable posture when considering exposure to AIDS. ALL EVIDENCE TO DATE INDICATES THAT BASIC INFECTION CONTROL PROCEDURES ARE MORE EFFECTIVE IN PREVENTING EXPOSURE TO AIDS THAN TO MOST OTHER DENTAL INFECTIOUS DISEASES.

The challenge to dentistry is not preventing AIDS. The challenge to dentistry is implementing disciplined, basic infection control procedures.

STRICT OBSERVANCE OF INFECTION CONTROL PROCEDURES WILL MINIMIZE RISKS OF ACQUIRING HIV AND OF CROSS-CONTAMINATION OF PATIENTS AND PERSONNEL. One bright light is that the HIV virus is quickly and easily inactivated[25] outside the body, and that such virus is very susceptible to efficacious disinfectants and sterilants. Even though the virus has been shown to be easily inactivated, a recent study by the Pasteur Institute in France has shown the HIV survives for UP TO 10 DAYS at room temperature outside the body.[26] They conclude:

> *This resistance [of the virus] at room temperature may explain the appearance of some AIDS cases in non-risk groups. To prevent possible contamination by viral particles in dry or liquid form, hygiene should be increased in the general population. Moreover, some more safety precautions should be taken in laboratories and in hospitals and BY DENTISTS who use a vacuum pump for saliva aspiration.*

INFECTION CONTROL PROCEDURES ARE PROVING TO BE VERY EFFECTIVE AGAINST THE AIDS VIRUS.

Other Emerging Diseases

Classic hepatitis B, herpes, and AIDS are not the only infectious diseases which must be of concern to dentistry. New emerging diseases, such as viral delta hepatitis, Creuzfeldt-Jakob Disease, legionellosis, and other presently more obscure diseases have the potential of evolving into seriousness in the wet finger environment.

Delta Hepatitis

Delta hepatitis virus (HDV) is an excellent example of an emerging and potentially very serious infectious disease. Reports of HDV have begun to appear more frequently in the literature and have been mentioned in the mass media. A recent editorial in the *New England Journal of Medicine*[27] titled "Delta Hepatitis—the Next Scourge?" stated:

During the past decade, a seemingly endless list of mysterious, newly described infectious diseases has captured the attention of the public. Now, just when you thought your imagination had been taxed to its limit, along comes the delta hepatitis virus.

Finally, although delta hepatitis can be prevented by vaccinating susceptible persons with hepatitis B vaccine, unfortunately, no simple method exists to protect hepatitis B carriers from delta superinfection. What will happen if delta is introduced into such hitherto spared groups with high frequencies of chronic hepatitis B as homosexual men or, as appears inevitable in today's world of global travel, Asian populations? Unless additional, intensive investigation of this novel agent and its properties provides clues to its control, we may be confronted with a new scourge.

HDV is a "piggy-back" virus which replicates only in persons who are already infected with active or carrier hepatitis B. DELTA HEPATITIS CANNOT OCCUR IN PERSONS WHO HAVE NATURAL OR ACQUIRED IMMUNITY TO VIRAL HEPATITIS B. Because there is no vaccine for delta, the only way to prevent acquiring the disease is to avoid becoming infected with hepatitis B. IN OTHER WORDS, IMMUNITY PROVIDED BY THE HBV VACCINES WILL ALSO PROTECT AGAINST DELTA HEPATITIS.

Delta hepatitis virus (HDV), originally called the delta agent, was discovered in 1977 by Rizzetto and colleagues in Italy.[28] Extensive investigations since that time have established the fact that delta hepatitis is unique and distinct from hepatitis B, although HDV is dependent upon hepatitis B virus (HBV) for clinical expression.[29] HDV is defective in that it requires HBV as a helper virus for an outer protein coat (HBsAg) and thus for replication.

HDV infection is worldwide in distribution and occurs in two major epidemiologic patterns. Delta is endemic in Mediterranean countries such as southern Italy, the Middle East and parts of Africa as it is in parts of South America. Nonpercutaneous transmission of HBV and HDV is believed to occur primarily by intimate contact and transmucosal exchange of body fluids.[30] In areas where HDV infection is nonendemic, including North America and Western Europe, HDV infection is confined to groups with frequent percutaneous exposures such as drug addicts and hemophiliacs. Preliminary studies in the United States have found HDV to be detectable in 24 percent of HBsAg positive drug addicts in the Los Angeles area[31] and approximately 50 percent of HBsAg positive hemophiliacs.[32] Studies indicate that about four percent of U.S. volunteer blood donors who are asymptomatic hepatitis B carriers are positive for either HDAg or anti-HD.[33] [34] Homosexual men, despite their high HBV infection rate, have been relatively spared HDV infection, although cases have been noted.[35]

Hepatitis relating to delta infection occurs in two primary ways.[36] The first mode is simultaneous infection with HBV and HDV. When simultaneous infection occurs, the acute clinical course of hepatitis often is limited with resolution of both hepatitis B and delta infections. The second mode involves acute delta infection in HBsAg carriers. In this situation the patient already has a high titer of circulating HBsAg. These patients are more likely to have a serious and possibly acute fulminant form of hepatitis that more often leads to chronic delta infection. Some of these patients will become carriers of HDV as well as HBsAg.

HDV has been associated with several U.S. hepatitis outbreaks. The largest outbreak, in Worcester, Massachusetts, is continuing with presently 408 total cases involving over 148 parenteral drug abusers. Over 65 of these individuals were positive for prior infection with HDV. There have been eleven deaths, eight of whom were delta positive. Three dentists have been infected through this outbreak to date (personal communication, Mr. Frank Birch).

As all dental staff members are at an increased risk of HBV infection and of possibly becoming hepatitis B carriers, members of the dental profession are at risk of simultaneous infection with

HDV and HBV. Additionally, it has been estimated there are currently 3,000 hepatitis B carriers in the dental profession in the U.S.[37] These individuals are also at risk of HDV super infection. Parenteral drug abusers infected with HDV are receiving routine dental treatment as many of these individuals do not report their recreational drug habits to the dentist.

The dental professional can prevent the clinical expression of delta infection by preventing a hepatitis B infection. Thus all dental personnel should wear masks, gloves and protective eyewear along with appropriate clinical attire in the daily treatment of *all* patients to protect themselves from HDV, HBV and other infectious agents carried by patients. In addition the dental professional can be protected by use of the hepatitis B vaccine.

All forms of hepatitis are a serious threat to members of the dental team; however, delta represents the most life threatening of these diseases. Dental personnel who are carriers, most of whom are unaware of their status, are most at risk for delta infection. Unfortunately, outbreaks of hepatitis B are becoming more numerous as is evident with the continuing outbreak in Worcester, Massachusetts, and the newly reported outbreak in Durham, North Carolina, with 86 cases of hepatitis, 15 percent of whom have markers for delta virus exposure. It behooves the dentist and his or her staff to take all precautions to prevent these preventable infections.

THE EXAMPLES OF THE SERIOUSNESS OF HEPATITIS NON-A, NON-B AND DELTA, HERPES II, AIDS, AND OTHER EMERGING DISEASES OF DENTAL CONCERN SHOULD SERVE AS CONSTANT REMINDERS THAT NEW, EMERGING DISEASES ARE CONTINUING THREATS TO THE SAFETY OF THE DENTAL ENVIRONMENT.

Summary

Dentistry is routinely challenged by a number of infectious diseases, and new diseases are expanding the list of diseases at a surprising rate.

Hepatitis B is still the most serious disease confronting the dental environment; however, acquired immunodeficiency syndrome (AIDS) is presently receiving nearly all of the media attention on infectious diseases. While it is very important to more fully understand AIDS, particularly in view of the front-line challenge to dentistry in potentially diagnosing the illness, it is also very important that personnel recognize the seriousness of other older and newer diseases in the dental environment.

If it was not for the public media's constant attention to AIDS, we would probably be reading more of infectious disease challenges to dentistry, for example viral delta hepatitis and the resurgence of tuberculosis in certain segments of society.

References and Suggested Readings

1. Isaacson, W., "Hunting for Hidden Killers," July 4, 1983, *Time*, 50-55.

2. Crawford, J. "State-of-the-Art: Practical Infection Control in Dentistry." JADA, 110:629-33, Apr, 1985.

3. University of Colorado News. "Dental School Sponsors Hepatitis Awareness Week." June, 1983.

4. Cottone, J., Goebel. "Hepatitis B: Detection and the Carrier Patient." Jnl of O S, O M, O P, 449-54, Oct, 1983.

5. Bond, Favero, *et al.* "Survival of Hepatitis B Virus After Drying and Storage for One Week." Lancet, 1:550-51, 1981.

6. Food and Drug Administration. "Safety of Hepatitis B Vaccine Confirmed." 15:2:14-15, Aug, 1985.

7. Laure, *et al.* "Hepatitis B Virus DNA Sequences in Lymphoid Cells from Patients with AIDS and AIDS-Related Complex." Science, 229:561-63, Aug, 1985.

8. American Dental Association. "Hepatitis B and the Dental Profession." Hepatitis Symposium, JADA, 110:614-50, Apr, 1985.

9. Manzella, *et al.* "An Outbreak of Herpes Simplex Virus Type I Gingivostomatitis in a Dental Hygiene Practice." JAMA, 252:15: 2019-22, Oct, 1984.

10. Molinari, J., *et al.* "Survival of Herpes Simplex Virus on Surfaces." Monitor, 1:1, Spring, 1984.

11. Loe, H., Johnson, S. "Herpes Vaccine in Animal Studies." JADA, 111:796, Nov, 1985.

12. Corey, L. "The Diagnosis and Treatment of Genital Herpes." JAMA, 248:9:1041-49, Sept, 1982.

13. Aurelian, L. "Possible Role of Herpesvirus Hominis, Type 2, in Human Cervical Cancer." Federation Proceedings, 31:6:1651-59, 1972.

14. Kibreck, S. "Herpes Simplex Infection at Term." JAMA, 243:2:157-60, Jan, 1980.

15. *The New York Times*, May 25, 1983.

16. Gallup, G. "Public Fears AIDS Will Spread." Gallup Poll, national media release, Aug 18, 1985.

17. Sivak, S., *et al.* "Estimated Number of Adults Infected with HTLV-III in the United States." N Engl Jnl Med, Nov 21, 1985.

18. Page, P. "AIDS Incubation Period." N Engl Jnl Med, 516, Aug 22, 1985.

19. Science News. "Cofactor in AIDS." 77, Aug 3, 1985.

20. Runnells, R.R., Ducel, G., *et al.* "Syndrome d'immunodeficience acqauise (SIDA)" from Runnells, R.R., RISQUE INFECTIEUX ET RESPONSABILITE AU CABINET DENTAIRE (Imprimerie Avenir SA, Geneva, Switz, 1984).

   Wofford, D., Miller, R. "AIDS: Disease Characteristics and Oral Manifestations." JADA, 111:258-61, Aug, 1985.

21. CDC. "Oral Viral Lesion Associated with AIDS." Morb and Mort Report, Sept 13, 1985.

22. *Ibid.*

23. *Ibid.*

24. Centers for Disease Control, "Healthcare Workers Contract AIDS," Morb & Mort Wkly Rprt, June 23, 1987.

25. Willett, N. "AIDS: Epidemiology, Biology and Significance to the Dental Profession." Calif Dent Assn Jnl, 27-34, Oct, 1985.

26. Chermann, *et al.* "Resistance of AIDS Virus at Room Temperature." Lancet, Sept 28, 1985.

27. Nishioka, N., Dienstag, J. "Delta Hepatitis: A New Scourge?" N Engl Jnl Med, 312:23:1515-16, June 6, 1985.

28. Rizzetto, M., and others. "Immunofluorescence detection of new antigen-antibody system (delta/anti-delta) associated to hepatitis B virus in liver and in serum of HBsAg carriers." (Gut 18:997-1003, 1977.

29. Rizzetto, M., and others. "Delta agent: association of delta antigen with hepatitis B surface antigen and RNA in serum of delta-infected chimpanzees." Proc Natl Acad Sci 77:6124-6128, 1980.

30. Friedman, L.S. and Dienstag, J.L. "Recent Developments in Viral Hepatitis." Yearbook Med Pub Inc., Chicago, 1986.

31. Govindarajan, S.; Kanel, G.C.; and Peters, R.L. "Prevalence of Delta-Antibody Among Chronic Hepatitis B-Virus Infected Patients in the Los Angeles Area. Its Correlation with Liver Biopsy Diagnosis." Gastroenterology 85:160, 1983.

32. Rizzetto, M.; Morello, C.; Na Mannucci, P.M., *et al.* "Delta Infection and Liver Disease in Hemophilic Carriers of the Hepatitis B Surface Antigen." J Inf Dis 145:18, 1982.

33. Mushahwar, I.K., and Dicker, R.H.: "Prevalence of Delta Antigen and Anti-Delta Detected by Immuno-Assays in Various HBsAg Positive Populations." The 1984 International Symposium on Viral Hepatitis, p. 23, 1984.

34. Nath, N., and others. "Antibodies to Delta Antigen in Asymptomatic Hepatitis B Surface Antigen-reactive Blood Donors in the United States and Their Association with Other Markers of Hepatitis B Virus." Am J Epidemiol 122(2):218-225, 1985.

35. Shields, M.T., *et al.* "Frequency and Significance of Delta Antibody in Acute and Chronic Hepatitis B. A United States Experience." Gastroenterology 89:1230-1235, 1985.

36. Cottone, J.A. "Delta Hepatitis: Another Concern for Dentistry." JADA 112:47-49, 1986.

37. Cottone, J.A. "Hepatitis B Virus Infection in the Dental Profession." JADA 110:617-621, 1985.

Chapter Four
REVIEW EXERCISES

Date _____Name_____

Circle the letters of the terms which most closely approximate the answers. There may be one or more than one correct answer. If you circle D, indicate the other answer or answers, if known.

1. Professional personnel are potentially exposed to:

    A. many virulent diseases   B. an occasional infection   C. a large number of pathogens

    D. other_____

2. Serious infectious diseases found in dentistry include:

    A. cardiotitis   B. hepatitis   C. AIDS

    D. other_____

3. Clinical (visible) diseases such as syphilis and herpes simplex are:

    A. not found in dentistry   B. the most serious of diseases C. resistant to sterilization

    D. other_____

4. Sub-clinical (invisible) diseases such as tuberculosis and pneumonia are:

    A. found in dentistry   B. easy to diagnose   C. less serious

    D. other_____

5. Emerging new diseases such as cytomegalovirus and AIDS are:

    A. not found in dentistry   B. venereal diseases only   C. the most difficult to diagnose

    D. other_____

6. Every time one disease is conquered:

A. it is controlled
indefinitely

B. the survival age increases

C. others evolve to seriousness

D. other_____

7. Potentially, the most serious emerging disease is:

A. AIDS

B. hepatitis

C. legionellosis

D. other_____

8. A common route of transmission of hepatitis B is:

A. saliva

B. blood

C. cut on fingers

D. other_____

9. Two vaccines have been developed for:

A. AIDS

B. herpes II

C. hepatitis

D. other_____

10. The causative factor of AIDS is:

A. a virus

B. a bacterium

C. unknown

D. other_____

11. An effective infection control program will automatically cope with:

A. AIDS

B. herpes

C. hepatitis

D. other_____

12. The impact of an infection control program on dental personnel affects:

A. compensation

B. continuing education

C. malpractice

D. other_____

13. Tuberculosis is:

   A. a dental threat   B. obsolete   C. potentially serious

   D. other_____

14. AIDS has infected:

   A. promiscuous gays   B. nurses   C. a dentist

   D. other_____

NOTE: Answers to the review questions appear in the back of this book.

The Dental Health Team and Patient Treatment

ABSTRACT: Infection control is a specialty within dentistry and is an evolving process which requires the same continuing attention as does cosmetic dentistry or caries prevention.

The classification of patients, through use of certain screening procedures, is a mandatory prerequisite to the practice of minimal, routine, or high risk infection control precautions.

Patients usually choose the services of a dentist and his staff because of the dentist's reputation, personality, technical skills, and/or office location. Few patients choose dental services because of the infection control procedures practiced in that office. Patients simply have "faith" that they will be protected from infection by qualified health professionals, and all dental personnel have an obligation not to violate that faith. Personnel can protect themselves, but patients can do little for protection except to depend on the honesty, dedication, and ability of professionals.

A dental practice is people, and perhaps the most important single consideration in establishing an effective infection control program is the hiring, training, and motivation of competent personnel. As with any other discipline, the product produced—in this case the control of infection—is only as good as the day-to-day workers on the production line.

Hiring and Motivating Personnel

Effective infection control requires special atten-
tion to minute detail. The discipline is exacting, at times highly repetitive, and not all persons are well suited to the work.

When hiring infection control personnel, dentists should look for persons who are mature, serious, somewhat introverted, meticulous in personal care, detail-oriented, prideful, and self-starting. They should be paid well, and they should be encouraged to make infection control a major interest. Minimum turn-over of personnel is a necessity to assure the continued effectiveness of a program.

Infection control is a process of continuous learning and, as such, requires the constant filtering and evaluating of new information and techniques. Staff must be motivated to help perform these functions. Motivation should be in the form of attractive compensation, generous fringe benefits, a comfortable and safe working environment, including protection from office-acquired infections, and a formalized continuing education program.

Compensation and benefits are determined by local competition for productive workers. Since dentistry is a relatively closed discipline in which dentists are sometimes not in contact with employers in other fields, dental wages and benefits may sometimes not be as attractive as those in industry. There are no bargains, and personnel must be fairly compensated if they are to be encouraged to make a career of practicing infection control of high quality.

Continuing education, paid for by the dentist, is a motivational tool nearly as important as compensation. The educational program should be diverse and should include seminars and courses in health, disease, microbiology, epidemiology, and other related sciences. Personnel should be encouraged to be active in infection control associations which cross disciplinary lines and which serve persons in medical, dental, microbiological, and related fields. Since the basics of infection control are the same in all fields, techniques used in one field, a medical office, may be adopted by another field, a dental office, with many advantages for patients and staff. A free exchange of information is very important.

INFECTION CONTROL IS AN EVOLVING EXACTING FIELD OF TECHNOLOGY, AND THE PROCESS IS UNENDING. NEW DISCOVERIES MAKE CHANGE MANDATORY IN ORDER TO TAKE ADVANTAGE OF STATE-OF-THE-ART ADVANCEMENTS.

Scientific periodicals should be provided to keep staff up-to-date with new techniques, advancements in science, and new products. Two excellent publications are the *Morbidity and Mortality Weekly Report* from the Superintendent of Documents, U.S. Government Printing Office, and *JORRI (The Journal of the Operating Room Research Institute).*[1] The *Report* gives the latest scientific information on infectious diseases. *JORRI* has excellent articles on practical advancements in a wide range of infection control procedures, and many manufacturers advertise new infection control products in *JORRI*. Other excellent publications include the *Journal of the American Dental Association, Applied Microbiology* and *Infection Control.*

CONTROL,[2] a dental infection control newsletter, should also be considered.

PERSONNEL MOTIVATION COMBINES CREATIVE INVOLVEMENT WITH MEANINGFUL ACCOMPLISHMENT, THEREBY CONTRIBUTING TO BETTER PATIENT AND FELLOW WORKER HEALTH.

Personnel Care and Hygiene

Patient protection begins with the personal concerns and hygiene of each member of the dental staff.

Clothing

In recent years, some dentists have begun to dress in casual street clothes when treating patients. The same dentists often require that staff also dress informally. A few dental clinicians have encouraged this informality to create a more relaxed dental environment. While there is some merit to the desire to relax patients, dressing casually does not meet the needs of an effective infection control program, and this informality may have the opposite effect on thoughtful patients. Imagine the reaction of an accident victim being wheeled into the emergency room of a hospital where the physicians are wearing sport shirts and slacks, and nurses are wearing jeans and sweaters. Certainly a dental office is not the emergency room of a hospital, but there are similar infection control considerations. Proper dress is important to a well-rounded infection control program.

Non-treatment staff may wear street clothing if desired, but all personnel working in patient treatment areas should wear freshly laundered professional uniforms.

Professional uniforms should be simple, as seamless as possible, and should have short sleeves. Studies[3] have shown that microorganisms accumulate on cuffs of long-sleeved uniforms following treatment. Since uniforms should be changed daily, they should be capable of withstanding frequent and multiple washings. Uniforms should be made of synthetic materials which retain fewer microbes and last longer than cotton fabrics. Uniforms should be kept at the office. Commuting on public transportation, or even in private autos, can soil or contaminate a fresh uniform. Wearing a uniform home at the end of a busy day may bring a multitude of unwanted microorganisms into an unsuspecting household, especially to susceptible children under one year of age. Changing to street clothes and carrying the uniform in a bag for laundering is a far more prudent tactic.

Uniforms should be freshly laundered, preferably by a commercial laundry. If uniforms are home laundered, they should be washed in a heavy-duty washing machine using strong detergent in hot water. Saliva spatters, water droplet aerosols, and blood accumulate, and studies have shown uniforms to be highly contaminated after limited use. A simple experiment of touching the surface of a uniform to an agar plate and culturing for 24 hours produces dramatic evidence of fabric contamination. (See Figure 1.)

IT MAKES LITTLE SENSE TO STERILIZE, DISINFECT, AND TREAT INSTRUMENTS AND WORK SURFACES AND YET WEAR CONTAMINATED CLOTHING.

Other clothing such as shoes and stockings should be simple and not ornate. Seams, buttons, buckles, and similar appendages should be avoided since they provide protection where microbes may accumulate and multiply.

Hair, Facial Hair and Jewelry

All treatment personnel should have short, well-managed hair. If long hair is occasionally a necessity, it must be kept in a bun or otherwise restrained or covered. In addition to the concern that long hair will brush contaminants into a patient treatment area, there is increased probability that stray or broken hairs will contaminate instruments or work surfaces. (See Figure 2.)

Beards and mustaches should be avoided by treatment personnel. Dental treatment creates an inordinate amount of droplets and splashes when compared to other health professions. Such vehicles can quickly transmit microorganisms to facial hair, often even when masks are worn.

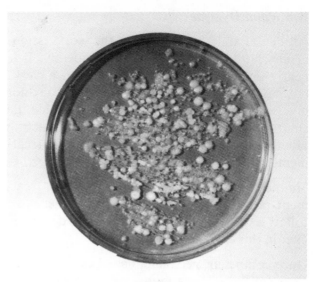

FIGURE 1
Growth of microorganisms from a soiled uniform touched to agar and cultured for 24 hours.

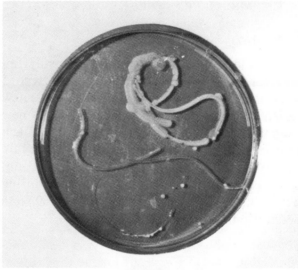

FIGURE 2
Human hair cultured on agar for 24 hours.

Jewelry, such as rings, watches, and bracelets, should not be worn by treatment staff. Jewelry offers protection to microbes and interferes with hand and arm washing. Additionally, mercury contamination of noble metal clasps can cause crystallization and breakage, with the possible loss of valuable gemstones.

Hand Hygiene

All dental staff, regardless of the work assignment, should wash their hands frequently. It is nearly impossible for a typist, insurance clerk, business office supervisor, or other persons not involved in treatment of patients to handle charts and other records without contacting saliva, blood, or other contaminants from treatment areas.

Simple handwashing is sufficient for non-treatment personnel, but treatment personnel must follow a specific washing technique, as described later in this chapter.

Once competent personnel have been trained in personal care, attention can be turned to improving an infection control program. All programs begin with screening and evaluation of patients.

Screening Patients

Patients seeking dental treatment normally fall into three categories: (1) Patients of record returning for regular or emergency care, (2) new patients seeking routine treatment, and (3) new patients seeking emergency treatment. Each group requires a special screening procedure before treatment to determine the infection control precautions which must be observed during treatment. (See Table 8 on pages 67 and 69 for a description of the precautions.)

Patients of Record

The last treatment date of a patient of record should be determined, and a new medical patient history should be taken on all patients not seen within a year or on a predetermined regular schedule. The medical history of all patients of record, regardless of when last seen, should be updated at each appointment. Any seriously questionable responses should be dealt with by postponing treatment until medical laboratory blood tests can be obtained and a treatment program can be planned.

In the absence of new significant information, previous patients of record, without a negative health profile, should be treated with routine infection control procedures.

New Routine Patients

New routine patients include non-emergency patients who are seeking routine dental care but who have not been previous patients of record. Most new routine patients will be seeking care voluntarily and, therefore, will be less likely to come from a high infection risk group.

Routine infection control procedures (outlined on the following pages) should be practiced unless the patient history profile identifies a reason for special concern. If reason for significant concern is identified, dental treatment should be postponed until medical laboratory tests can be obtained and the results evaluated to detect the presence of infection, such as hepatitis B.

Emergency Patients

Emergency patients of record who have been treated recently should have routine care, but emergency patients not of record should be screened very carefully, since many high risk groups such as drug users often neglect their dental health and seek mainly emergency treatment.

Many high risk groups seek emergency dental care for oral symptoms resulting from serious infection. For example, AIDS patients may seek dental treatment for herpes simplex, candidiasis, or Kaposi's sarcoma—all symptomatic of AIDS infection.[4]

Since new emergency patients must be considered potentially high infection risks, special infection control precautions should be practiced, and only absolutely necessary relief procedures should be performed until the results of all medical questions and tests are received and evaluated. Staff protection measures must be rigidly observed.

Many emergency patients become excellent

patients of record who contribute to the growth of a practice, but the high risk potential of this group must not be ignored in a desire to "cultivate" patients.

Patient History

As a part of the screening process, a complete patient history must be taken on all new and certain former patients of record, as previously described. The purpose of the patient history is to secure information necessary for dental treatment and to construct a profile useful in determining whether high risk infection control precautions are to be observed during treatment.

Patient histories are valuable aids in the identification of high risk patients. However, studies have shown that patients do not always answer health-related questions truthfully. Drug users and homosexuals—two high infection risk groups—may be reluctant to admit their personal habits. Also, infective carriers are not always aware that they harbor disease. A recent study of dental school patients showed that of twenty-two patients who tested positive to hepatitis B, only four were aware of or would admit to the disease.[5]

Even with possible distortions of patient history information, such histories are absolutely necessary. The confidential history questionnaire should be designed to provide a patient profile and should include, in addition to the usual family, work, and other routine queries, very specific questions pertaining to disease, such as:

1. When was the last time you had a blood test?

2. Have you ever had a blood transfusion?

3. Have you ever had a renal dialysis?

4. Have you ever been told you are a carrier of a disease—for example, hepatitis?

5. Have you ever been near someone with hepatitis?

6. Have you ever had liver problems or jaundice?

7. Do you have leukemia or hemophilia?

8. Have you ever had a lingering illness? What kind?

9. Have you ever been treated for drug-related problems?

10. Have you ever been out of the United States? Where?

11. Do you have any allergies?

12. Have you had a noticeable loss of memory?

Other questions should be developed and should include those which may help to identify specific diseases of special local prevalence—for example, AIDS prone homosexuals and drug users, and "Third World" immigrants.

Unstable political and socio-economic conditions in many Caribbean, Latin American, and Southeast Asian countries have caused a high influx of immigrants to the United States. Many of these people have had little health care, and they are highly susceptible to certain pathogens. Although international health organizations attempt to screen most immigrants, some disease carrying individuals escape detection. There has been a substantial increase in the United States of certain diseases, such as tuberculosis and leprosy, that were once thought to be nearly eradicated.

If some patients object to answering personal questions, it should be explained that the information is needed to better protect them and dental office staff from cross-contamination. When they will not volunteer information, special high risk precautions should be exercised during treatment. It is highly desirable to have such patients' blood tested by a medical laboratory for hepatitis and other potential infective agents before treatment. One of the reasons patients may refuse to divulge information is that they may suspect they are harboring disease, and they wish to resist recognizing the problem.

The patient questionnaire should be carefully evaluated BEFORE treatment is begun. If the profile is suspect, treatment should be postponed until medical laboratory results are received and evaluated.

A sample comprehensive patient evaluation questionnaire is shown on the following two pages.

Preventive Measures

There are a number of precautionary and preventive procedures which are necessary for the control of infection. At least a minimal precautionary program for infection control must always be practiced. As personnel become better trained in control, an optimum, or routine, program should be adopted. When treating high risk patients, personnel must unfailingly practice a special high risk program. A summary chart of the three suggested programs is presented later in this chapter.

Routine Program

The following routine preventive measures should be observed when treating all patients:

1. The dental receptionist should routinely ask all patients how they are feeling and report any negative response to the dentist. If there is a question about the health of a patient, treatment should be postponed until further information is secured.

2. Patients should rinse their mouths with an antimicrobial mouthwash before treatment. This action has been shown to reduce the number of oral microbes by up to ninety percent but does not replace other precautions.

3. Personnel should use rubber gloves for all procedures possible, especially when the fingers or hands are cut or nicked. TWO COUNCILS OF THE AMERICAN DENTAL ASSOCIATION RECOMMEND WEARING OF GLOVES FOR THE TREATMENT OF ALL PATIENTS. If full gloving is not possible, at least rubber fingercots should be used to cover injured or sensitive fingers. Non-sterile gloves are less expensive and may be worn for the making of routine examinations, the taking of x-rays, and the performing of most treatment procedures on all new or emergency patients, the goal of gloving in these procedures being to protect staff and patients from cross-contamination. Sterile gloves should always be worn for invasive procedures, since protection of the patient from foreign tissue infection is the goal.

While the use of gloves is common in certain disciplines in dentistry, such as oral surgery, gloving is relatively new to most general practitioners.

Resistance is not unusual based on the need for "tactile sense." It is of interest that the same objections were raised when gloving was introduced to medical surgery in the 1890s. Training and habit has eliminated the excuse in medicine, where delicate surgery is performed routinely.

A review of glove basics may help personnel to avoid certain problems. Gloves are manufactured from two types of materials, latex and vinyl. Vinyl gloves are generally used by health professionals only for certain non-treatment procedures, but vinyl is normally not considered an acceptable material for treatment gloves because of its lack of elasticity and its lower tensile strength.

Latex is the preferred material for gloves. It is used in the manufacture of a number of types of gloves, including examination, surgical, anatomical, ambidextrous, procedure, multi-purpose, utility, and housekeeping. The needs of dentistry can usually be satisfied by the use of three types of gloves—non-sterile exam, sterile ambidextrous surgical, and a utility or housekeeping type—and fingercots.

The cost difference between a superior and an average glove is only a matter of one or two cents, and the quality of glove is so critical that only the best should be used. The difference in cost is determined mostly by the manufacturing process. Certain gloves are made by the "coagulation" process whereby the gloves are formed by the dipping of a mold one time into latex after the mold has been coated with a

PATIENT EVALUATION QUESTIONNAIRE

MARK EACH CIRCLE COMPLETELY FOLLOWING EACH QUESTION AND COMPLETE APPROPRIATE ANSWERS.

Name _____
(Last, First, Middle)

Address _____
(Number and Street)   (City, State, Zip)

How long at present address? 0-1 year ○   1-3 years ○   3 years or more ○

Home Phone _____ Business Phone _____

Former Address _____
(Number and Street)   (City, State, Zip)

Date of Birth_____ Sex_____ Height_____ Weight_____ Occupation_____ Employer_____

Social Security No. _____-_____-_____   Single ○   Divorced ○   Married: 0-2 years ○ 2-5 years ○ 5+ years ○   Children: ○ Yes ○ No

Name of Spouse_____ Closest Relative _____ Phone_____

Referred By _____ Physician_____ Phone_____

Insurance Company_____ Policy Number_____

GENERAL:

1.   Are you a U.S. citizen? . . . . ○ Yes   ○ No

2.   If not a citizen, when did you enter the U.S.?_____

     From what country?_____

3.   Have you visited another country in the last three years? . . . . ○ Yes   ○ No

     If so, where and when?_____ For how long: 2 weeks or less ○ 2-10 weeks ○ Longer ○

4.   Have you ever been seriously ill in another country? . . . . ○ Yes   ○ No

     If so, what was the illness?_____

5.   Have you ever participated in the Peace Corps, foreign educational exchange, or other exchange program or occupation? . . . . . . ○ Yes   ○ No

     If so, what country(ies)?_____

6.   Do you presently work in a healthcare facility? . . . . ○ Yes   ○ No

     If so, do you care for patients? . . . . ○ Yes   ○ No

7.   Do you presently work in an institution? . . . . ○ Yes   ○ No

8.   Have you ever worked in a hospital, institution, microbiological or testing laboratory? . . . . ○ Yes   ○ No

     If so, when and what type facility?_____

9.   Have you been in the armed forces in the last three years? . . . . ○ Yes   ○ No

     If so, where?   U.S. ○   Overseas ○

10. Do you presently live in a retirement center or nursing home? . . . . ○ Yes   ○ No

DENTAL:

11. Do you have any of the following in/on your mouth, tongue, lips, or neck? (If yes, mark circle.)

A.	New swelling in mouth.	○	F.	Cold sores.	○
B.	Swollen, purplish gums.	○	G.	Swollen glands on neck.	○
C.	Grey-white rash on cheek or tongue.	○	H.	Bleeding gums.	○
D.	Grey-white growth on side of tongue.	○	I.	Other problems.	○
E.	Canker sores.	○	J.	If you checked any of the above, when did you first notice symptoms?	

_____

12. Have you had unusual bleeding with previous extractions or surgery? . . . . ○ Yes   ○ No

13. Are your teeth painful? . . . . ○ Yes   ○ No

14. Can you chew on both sides of your mouth? . . . . ○ Yes   ○ No

15. How often do you brush your teeth?_____

PLEASE COMPLETE REVERSE SIDE OF THIS QUESTIONNAIRE

MEDICAL:

16. Are you presently under the care of a physician? . . . . ○ Yes   ○ No

    If so, why?_____

17. Have you been a patient in a hospital in the past three years? . . . . ○ Yes   ○ No

    If so, what were you treated for?_____

18. Have you been in any other institution (weight reduction, drug or alcohol treatment, mental, psychiatric, or other) in the last three years? . . . . ○ Yes   ○ No

    If so, which one(s)?_____

19. Have you had a blood transfusion in the past three years? . . . . ○ Yes   ○ No

20. Do you perspire excessively at night? . . . . ○ Yes   ○ No

21. Do you have persistent diarrhea? . . . . ○ Yes   ○ No

22. Have you lost weight recently without dieting? . . . . ○ Yes   ○ No

    How many pounds?   Less than 10 ○   10-30 ○   Over 30 ○

23. Do you have a purplish rash or persistent purplish bruise(s)? . . . . ○ Yes   ○ No

24. Are you presently taking any of the following medicine or treatment drugs? . . . . ○ Yes   ○ No
    Please mark exact drug(s).

IMURAN	○	DELTASONE	○	CYCLOSPORINE ○	PREDNISONE ○
PURIMETHOL	○	CORTICOSPORINE	○	CORTICOSTEROIDS ○	HYDROCORTISONE ○
CYTOXAN	○	DECADRON	○	STEROIDS ○	
METHOTREXATE	○	METACORTEN	○	CORTISONE ○	

    If not listed, name other drug(s) you are taking: _____

25. Do you occasionally take recreational drugs? . . . . ○ Yes   ○ No

    How often?_____

26. Are you allergic to any drugs or medicine? . . . . ○ Yes   ○ No

    If so, which one(s)?_____

27. Have you ever had any excessive bleeding requiring special treatment? . . . . ○ Yes   ○ No

28. Have you had prolonged coughing or coughed up blood? . . . . ○ Yes   ○ No

29. Have you ever had a blood test for hepatitis or AIDS? . . . . ○ Yes   ○ No

    Results were: Negative (no virus) ○   Positive (virus present) ○

30. If so, were you vaccinated? . . . . ○ Yes   ○ No

31. Have you had cankers, cold sores or other sores on your lips, tongue, gums, genitals, or body in the past three years? . . . . ○ Yes   ○ No

32. Circle any of the following which you have had or now have:
    (If so, put date to the left of the letter marked.)

A.	AIDS ○	J.	chronic cough ○	S.	jaundice ○
B.	allergies ○	K.	diabetes ○	T.	kidney treatment ○
C.	anemia ○	L.	epilepsy ○	U.	organ transplant ○
D.	arthritis ○	M.	heart murmur ○	V.	psychiatric treatment ○
E.	artificial heart valves ○	N.	heart trouble ○	W.	shortness of breath ○
F.	asthma ○	O.	hepatitis ○	X.	sinus trouble ○
G.	cancer treatment ○	P.	herpes ○	Y.	stroke ○
H.	cardiac pacemaker ○	Q.	high blood pressure ○	Z.	swelling of ankles ○
I.	congenital heart lesions ○	R.	HIV virus ○	AA.	tuberculosis ○
				BB.	venereal disease ○

33. Have you had any other serious illnesses? . . . . ○ Yes   ○ No

34. If female, are you pregnant now? . . . . ○ Yes   ○ No

35. If female, are you nursing? . . . . ○ Yes   ○ No

    TO BE ANSWERED ONLY BY PATIENTS RECEIVING SEDATION OR GENERAL ANESTHESIA—

36. Have you had anything to eat or drink within the last 4 hours? . . . . ○ Yes   ○ No

37. Are you wearing removable dental appliances? . . . . ○ Yes   ○ No

38. Are you wearing contact lenses? . . . . ○ Yes   ○ No

39. Do you have someone to drive you home today? . . . . ○ Yes   ○ No

Signature _____

Reviewed By _____ Date_____

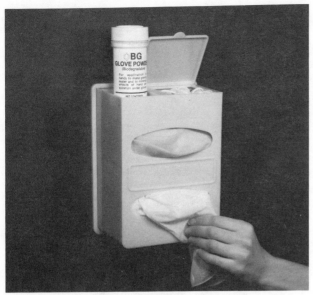

FIGURE 3
Glove dispenser holds two sizes of gloves, cots and glove powder.

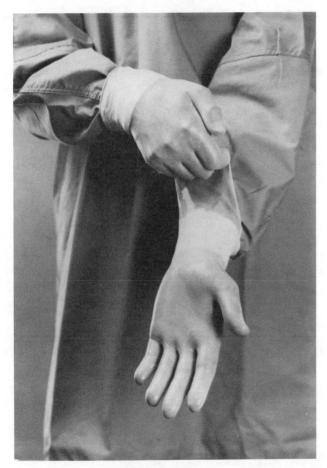

FIGURE 4
Examination gloves.

catalyzing coagulent. This process may leave chemical irritants in the gloves which can irritate skin and, since the process single dips in latex, the chance for pin holes is greater. Of course, pin holes may allow microorganisms to penetrate the glove and defeat the purpose for the gloving. A preferable glove is one that has been made by the "straight dip" process where the glove is dipped twice in latex and then vulcanized. No potentially irritating coagulant is used, and the double dipping process assures fewer pin holes and imperfections.

Gloves are coated with either cornstarch or talcum powder to facilitate handling and to minimize skin irritation. Whenever possible, only cornstarch coating should be used since it is an organic material which is absorbed by tissue. Talcum is inorganic and may interfere with tissue healing if left in an open wound.

Wherever possible, only latex straight dip gloves (not coagulant types) with cornstarch coating should be used. Gloves should be kept organized and readily accessible.

Gloves and cots should be conveniently located, and all necessary sizes should be

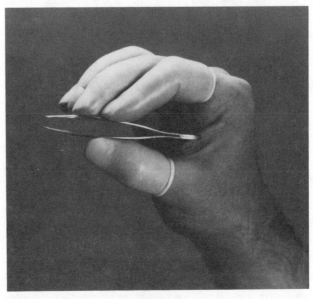

FIGURE 5
Fingercots for covering punctures or nicks when full gloving is not possible.

59

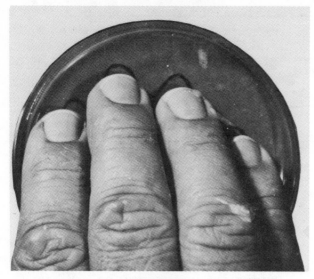

FIGURE 6
Dirty fingers touch agar.

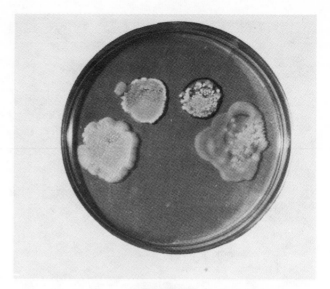

FIGURE 7
After 24-hour incubation.

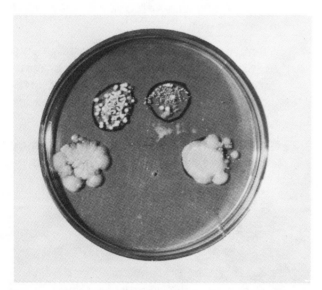

FIGURE 8
After cold water rinse.

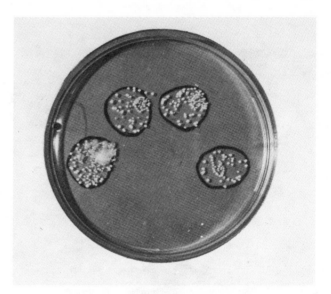

FIGURE 9
After 20-second wash with soap and water.

available. Hiding gloves in drawers often discourages use by some personnel.

4. Hands should be washed before treating patients and during treatment, as indicated. Hands should be washed, even if gloves are worn, to avoid the transporting of contamination to other areas. It is not possible or practical to maintain hospital surgical asepsis in dental treatment areas. Therefore, it is not necessary to use a "surgical scrub" technique when washing hands. The first wash in the morning, after lunch, and after the last patient should include scrubbing with a sterile or disinfected hand brush. Since scrubbing may occasionally result in abrasions and breaks in the skin or under the nails, brushing should be used when necessary only for removal of gross dirt and debris from the hands. Once gross dirt removal has been accomplished, quick,

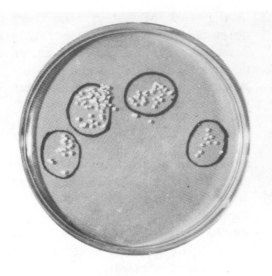

FIGURE 10
After additional 20-second wash with soap and water.

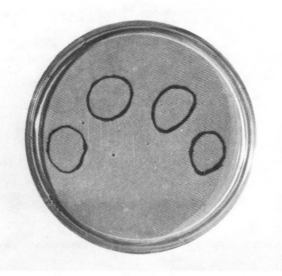

FIGURE 11
After using antimicrobial solution.

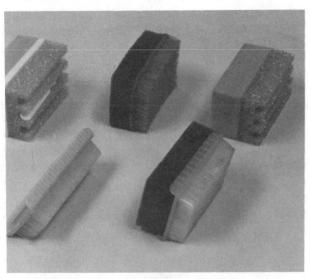

FIGURE 12
Examples of disposable and disinfectable brushes.

multiple washing and rinsing is most effective in reducing microbial count. Between patients, hands should be lathered and rinsed quickly three times, but fifteen seconds each time. The goal of the between patient hand wash is to remove transient pathogens which have adhered to the hands during patient treatment. Resident microbes normally found on hands of treatment personnel are not usually pathogenic and are not a major concern.

Studies have shown that the wash-rinse-wash-rinse-wash-rinse technique between patients is an effective way of reducing to a manageable level the numbers of transient microbes on the hands.[6]

The University of Georgia, College of Agriculture, has studied handwashing extensively.[7] Their work dramatically emphasizes the value of multiple washing and the use of an antimicrobial soap. PCMX's, chlorhexidines, and iodophors are acceptable soap chemicals. (See Figures 6-11.)

The agar plates illustrated were incubated for microbial growth following the hand treatment described under each figure.

Inexpensive disposable hand brushes, impregnated with a biocidal soap, are available and should be used when it is not possible to effectively disinfect or sterilize brushes. Brushes with sharp bristles should be avoided. Brushes with rounding bristle tips should be used to protect the hands from minute cuts and abrasions. Brushes should be stored in fresh disinfectant between patients and discarded when soiled and after use on any suspected high risk patient. Unfortunately, the only readily available resterilizable brushes are of the

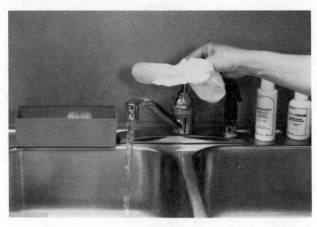

FIGURE 13
Turning faucet off with paper towel prevents recontamination.

stiffer nylon type and can abrade or cut hands and fingers.

5. Fingernails should be short and should be cleaned with an orange wood stick, rounded plastic, or similar device. A knife or sharp pointed instrument should not be used because breaking or cutting of the skin under the nails may result. Fingernails should always be cleaned and scrubbed before leaving the office at night. It has been shown that pathogens can be protected for many days under fingernails.

6. If the office is equipped with standard hand-actuated faucets, the handles should be disinfected between patients. Additionally, water should be left running after handwashing until the hands are dried with a disposable paper towel. Before discarding the towel, the faucet should be turned off using the towel as a barrier between the faucet handle and the hands. This simple step helps prevent re-contamination of the hands. (See Figure 13.)

7. While the three-wash-three-rinse handwashing technique is the most important part of microbial reduction on the hands, it is also desirable to use a disinfecting soap. Soaps containing PCMX, chlorhexidine gluconate or iodophors are effective, although sometime drying to the skin. Although soaps containing hexachlorophene are also available, there is evidence

in the work of certain researchers that potential toxicity may occur. Also, hexachlorophenes may build a bacteriostatic film on hands with multiple washings. Another disadvantage of hexachlorophene is that it is inactivated by alcohol.

Personnel with sensitive skin may find it desirable to use a mild emollient lotion after washing. If continuous use of the antimicrobial soap irritates hands, periodic use of a non-microbial milder soap is acceptable. However, microbial soap should always be used for the first and last wash of the day and whenever high risk patients are being treated.

It is also highly desirable to leave an antimicrobial residue on the hands after washing. The Association of Operatory Room Nurses cites this need as one of the three main objectives of handwashing.[8] For staff whose hands peel or crack with repeated washing, a single quick washing between patients, followed by application of an antimicrobial cream is acceptable. The cream has been found to be effective in controlling microbes. Cream should not be used routinely in place of the triple wash-rinse technique or when treating high risk patients. An interesting device, Nebucid, has recently been introduced in Europe. (See Figure 14.) The device nebulizes a liquid disinfectant onto the hands and dramatically reduces the number of microbes.

8. All soap and lotion dispensers should be wall hung and should be actuated only with the foot or forearm. Hands should be dried only with disposable paper towels dispensed from a "no touch" dispenser. The use of hot air driers has been suggested for dentistry, but the cost of the initial unit and the uncertainty of future energy costs make the use of such units questionable. CLOTH TOWELS SHOULD NOT BE USED UNLESS ABSOLUTELY NECESSARY AND THEN SHOULD BE USED ONLY ONCE.

9. Rubber dam should be used during all operative procedures to isolate the saliva

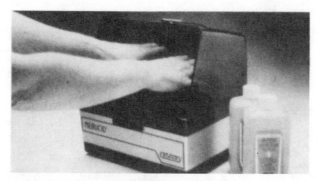

FIGURE 14
Nebucid hand disinfector nebulizes disinfectant onto hands to kill microbes.

and to retract the tissues to avoid tissue injury and subsequent bleeding. Saliva and blood, without proper isolation, may be spread by handpiece aerosol droplets, syringe splashes, and fingers. The Centers for Disease Control investigated the spread of hepatitis B by airborne aerosol transmission and concluded that "true airborne transmission of hepatitis B from infectious blood or saliva is not likely."[9] Airborne aerosol should not be confused with handpiece aerosol, where droplets of blood and saliva are generated. Handpiece aerosol is potentially infective.

10. Effective high volume evacuation (HVE) should be used to limit the aerosol droplets and splatter whenever the handpiece and syringe are used.

11. Eye protection or face shields should be worn by all personnel when treating patients, whether or not they are needed for corrective vision, to reduce the possibility of handpiece aerosol droplets and splatters entering the eyes. The Centers for Disease Control studied eye infection in a chimpanzee, in which systemic hepatitis B was induced nine weeks after the infecting of the eye of the animal with plasma from a hepatitis B patient.[10] The eyes can be a source of many infections.

Consideration should be given to covering patients' eyes during certain treatment, particularly when using the highspeed handpiece. Splashes, splatters, or aerosol droplets may enter patients' eyes during procedures, thereby leading to infection.

12. All personnel should wear masks at all times when treating patients, and masks should be changed frequently, preferably after each patient. Masks are available which are comfortable and which can be worn continuously without limiting breathing. Some masks are more efficacious than others,[11] and those offering the best filtration and most comfort should be used.

13. Treatment personnel should always wash their hands before and after handling patient records.

Disinfection, sterilization, and certain other control procedures are discussed in more detail in other chapters.

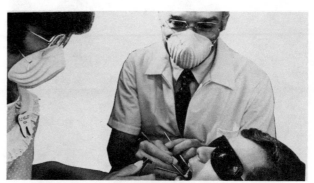

FIGURE 15
Protective glasses and preferred dome type mask.

Special Precautions

Infection control procedures must not be compromised in the treatment of HIGH RISK patients. In addition to the routine procedures listed above, the following precautions must be followed when treating HIGH RISK patients:

1. In addition to a complete patient history, medical laboratory blood tests should be required. Treatment should be postponed until the results of such tests are received and evaluated.

2. All dental personnel involved in direct patient care should be vaccinated for high risk diseases, such as hepatitis B, before treating patients.

Dental staff treating medically compromised patients should consider being vaccinated for all diseases possible, such as measles, rubella, flu and others to prevent the transmission of such diseases to the weakened patients.

3. Gloves must be worn by all treatment personnel at all times and must be discarded following treatment.

4. Disposable gowns should be used to minimize the possibility of contamination of the next patient and to minimize cross-contamination of staff.

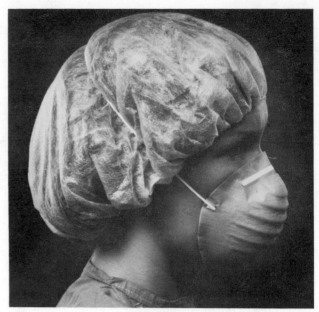

FIGURE 17
Disposable hair cover and preferred dome type face mask.

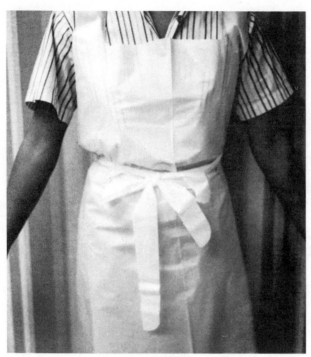

FIGURE 16
Protective disposable apron.

5. Disposable hair covers should be used by treatment staff and should be discarded immediately after treatment. Aerosols coat hair with contaminants.

6. All waste must be containerized, sealed, and disposed of immediately after treatment, preferably by incineration.

7. All contaminated instruments should be sterilized BEFORE cleaning, then cleaned and sterilized a SECOND TIME.

8. All surfaces, equipment, and items in or near the treatment area should be disinfected TWICE by using a maximum of disinfecting sponges generously saturated with fresh disinfectant.

9. Disposable drapes should be used to cover the chair and as many other surfaces as it is practical to cover. Removal of equipment from the treatment area minimizes the need to cover or disinfect it.

10. Dental units, cuspidors, and the HVE system should be flushed with fresh water for ten minutes immediately following treatment. Disinfectant should be circulated through the evacuation system and left as long as possible, preferably at least thirty minutes, before the treatment of the next patient.

11. Personnel should shower when possible or at least wash their hands, arms, faces, and ears with an antimicrobial soap immediately following treatment. A biocidal residual should be left on skin following washing.

12. Eyeglasses should be washed thoroughly and disinfected following treatment.

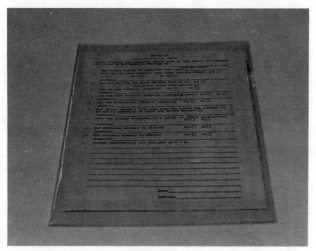

FIGURE 18
Patient chart in protective plastic cover.

13. Patient charts, records, and x-rays should be placed in disposable, transparent covers before use in the treatment area, and the covers should be discarded immediately following treatment. Only those records necessary in treatment should be in the treatment area.

14. Pencils and pens should never be placed near the mouth. Writing instruments should be disinfected, or sterilized if possible, as is done with any other instrument.

15. There should be as little physical contact between high risk patients and personnel as possible.

See tables on the next two pages for additional procedures.

Some of the above precautions may initially seem to be exaggerated, but it must be realized that high risk patients are potentially as dangerous to dental personnel as diseased patients are to medical hospital personnel. When treating high risk patients, dental office personnel must simulate as many hospital infection control procedures as possible.

In conclusion, various groups of patients offer varying degrees of exposure to pathogenic organisms. Screening patients before treatment provides a profile that helps dentists to determine which procedures and precautions must be observed in the treatment of each patient. In this way, dental staff can provide effective infection control that minimizes the possibility of cross-contamination.

Table 8 on the next two pages summarizes three suggested programs of infection control precautions, a choice of one of which should be observed when treating different types of patients.

References and Suggested Readings

1. The Journal of Operating Room Research Institute, 100 Campus Road, Totowa, New Jersey 07512.

2. I.C. Publications, 1150 East Nicholls Road, Fruit Heights, Utah 84037.

3. Williams, Shay, *et al.* "Indications of the Sanitation Level in a Dental Clinic," 1976, J Balt Coll Dent Surg, 31:1.

4. Cooley and Lubow. "AIDS: An Occupational Hazard?" July, 1983, Jnl of Am Dent Assoc, Vol 107:28-31.

5. Tullman, Boozer, *et al.* "The Threat of Hepatitis B from Dental School Patients," March, 1980. Oral Surg, Vol 49:3:214-216.

6. "An Evaluation of Surgical Scrubs in the Dental Clinic." Military Med, May, 1978, 347-348.

7. Schuler, Christian, *et al.* "Foods, Hands and Bacteria," March, 1980. Bulletin, 693.

8. "Standards for Surgical Hand Scrubs," May, 1976. Assoc of Oper Rm Nurs Jnl, 976.

9. Bond, M.S. "Viral Hepatitis B: Safety in the Immuno Chemistry Laboratory," 1982, Liqand Qtrly, 5:1:34-39.

10. Bond, Peterson, *et al.* "Transmission of B Hepatitis Via Eye Innoculation of a Chimpanzee," March, 1982. Jnl of Clin Microb, 533-534.

11. Clinical Research Associates Newsletter, "Surgical Face Masks," March, 1983, 7:3:1.

The Table on the reverse of this page is designed to be placed on the wall or other surface as a constant reminder of information which might be otherwise forgotten.

It is suggested that the Table be placed in a protective plastic cover or plastic laminate before being affixed to the wall or surface.

TABLE 8
TREATMENT PROCEDURE REMINDERS FOR
ROUTINE - RISK - HIGH RISK PATIENTS

PROCEDURE	ROUTINE	RISK	HIGH RISK
1. Personnel Vaccination, Especially HBV	Yes	Yes	MANDATORY
2. Wear Latex Exam Gloves	Yes	Always	DOUBLE-GLOVING
3. Wear Fingercots	In emergency only	No. Gloving only.	MANDATORY DOUBLE GLOVING
4. Wash With Long-Acting Microbial Soap	Yes	Hands, face, arms, and all exposed skin	SHOWER IF POSSIBLE
5. Use Soft, Non-Abrasive Handbrushes	Yes	Yes	Yes
6. Wear Fresh, Short-Sleeved Uniforms	Yes, change daily	Yes, change after each treatment	MANDATORY Disposable Gowns and Hair Covers
7. Wear Aprons Between Treatment Areas and Laboratory	Yes	Disposable aprons only	MANDATORY Disposable aprons ONLY
8. Wear Protective Eyeglasses	Yes	Yes, wash and disinfect after treatment	MANDATORY Wash and Disinfect by Immersion
9. Wear Protective Masks	Yes, at all times during treatment	Yes, and discard after treatment	MANDATORY Discard. Surgically Effective Filter Mask Should be Worn Under the Dome Mask
10. Wear Short, Well-Managed Hair; Avoid Facial Hair	Yes	Yes	Yes
11. Use of Cloth Towels	Should not be re-used in patient treatment	Use disposable paper towels only	DISPOSABLE TOWELS ONLY
12. Avoid Touching Sinks, Taps, Etc., Without Using A Barrier	Yes	Use "No-Touch" technique	MUST DISINFECT AND COVER WITH A BARRIER MANDATORY
13. Patients Rinse Mouth With Antimicrobial Mouthwash Before Treatment	Yes	Yes	MANDATORY Before and During Treatment
14. Use Rubber Dam for All Procedures	Yes	MANDATORY	MANDATORY
15. Use High Volume Evacuation on All Patients	Yes and discard HVE Tip after each use	Yes, and flush 1 or 2 minutes after treatment with HVE cleaner and disinfect, then discard tip	MANDATORY Disposable Tip Must Be Discarded. After Treatment, Flush HVE for At Least 10 Minutes
16. Clean-Up Personnel Wear Unlined Latex Utility Gloves When Handling Contaminated Instruments	Yes	Latex only, and should be washed and disinfected	MANDATORY LATEX GLOVES USED AND DISCARDED
17. Contaminated Instruments Stored in Holding Solution	Yes	Yes, fresh and of maximum strength	YES, MUST BE FRESH AND MAXIMUM STRENGTH
18. Instruments, Etc. Always Cleaned in Ultrasonic Cleaner	Yes	Yes, solution should be fresh and discarded immediately after use	SOLUTION MUST BE FRESH AND DISCARDED IMMEDIATELY AFTER USE
19. Sterilized Everything in Heat or Heat/Pressure Sterilizer	Yes, wherever possible	Yes, Before and after cleaning	MANDATORY Before and after cleaning

TABLE 8
TREATMENT PROCEDURE REMINDERS FOR
ROUTINE - RISK - HIGH RISK PATIENTS

PROCEDURE	ROUTINE	RISK	HIGH RISK
20. Circulate Water through Water Outlets	Yes, each morning and 15 seconds between each treatment	MANDATORY Flush 15 seconds after each treatment	MANDATORY FLUSH ONE MINUTE AFTER EACH TREATMENT
21. Disinfect Items When Sterilization Not Possible	Yes, all items possible	Yes, fresh disinfectant only. Barrier preferred.	USE DISPOSABLE BARRIERS ONLY
22. Practice Quality Assurance Sterilization Procedures	Yes	Use biological monitors weekly rather than monthly	USE BIOLOGICAL MONITORS EACH LOAD
23. Complete Quality Assurance Checklist	Yes	MANDATORY	MANDATORY
24. Use Barrier Coverings on Equipment and Surfaces	Yes, whenever practical	Yes, disposable barriers when possible	DISPOSABLE BARRIERS MUST BE USED ON ALL SURFACES POSSIBLE
25. Use Disposable Items When Possible	Yes	Yes	MANDATORY—MAXIMUM
26. Divide Bulk Packaged Items for Single	Yes	Yes, discard any remaining items	YES, MUST DISCARD ANY REMAINING ITEMS
27. Instruments and Items Should Be Pre-Packaged	Yes	Yes, clean and resterilize any remaining items	YES, STERILIZE ANY REMAINING ITEMS BEFORE USE
28. Required Patient Records for Patient Treatment in Treatment Area Only	Yes, handle only with freshly washed hands	Yes, in disposable plastic covers	YES, MUST BE COVERED WITH DISPOSABLE PLASTIC COVER AND DISCARDED AFTER PATIENT TREATMENT
29. Rinse and Spray All X-Ray Packets	Yes	Yes, immediately after treatment	MANDATORY AFTER TREATMENT
30. Dispose of Contaminated Waste Daily	Yes, preferably by incineration	Yes, place in plastic bags, seal (sterilized), discard outside office	MUST PLACE IN PLASTIC BAGS, SEAL, STERILIZED, DISCARD OUTSIDE OFFICE
31. Pumice Changed and Disinfected Daily	Yes	Dispose of immediately after treatment	DISPOSE OF IMMEDIATELY AFTER TREATMENT AND DISINFECT TRAY, ETC.
32. Items Used in Mouths Cleaned and Disinfected before Handling	Yes	Yes, with fresh disinfectant only	YES, INCREASING TIME TO 20 MINUTES
33. Disinfect Items Used on Dental Lathe	Yes, after each use	Yes, with fresh disinfectant	YES, WITH FRESH DISINFECTANT. STERILIZE IF POSSIBLE.
34. Contaminated Equipment Disinfected	Yes, between patient treatment	Yes, with fresh disinfectant	COVER WITH DISPOSABLE BARRIERS, THEN DISCARD AND DISINFECT SURFACES
35. Mark Packages Sent To Commercial Laboratories ''Caution''		MANDATORY, WITH FOLLOW-UP TELEPHONE CALL	MANDATORY, WITH FOLLOW-UP TELEPHONE CALL
36. High Risk Cases Scheduled at End of Day			MANDATORY
37. Remove Unnecessary Equipment from Treatment Room Before Treating High Risk Patients			MANDATORY
38. Postpone Treatment of High Risk Patient If Health Improvement Evident			MANDATORY

The Table on the reverse of this page is designed to be placed on the wall or other surface as a constant reminder of information which might be otherwise forgotten.

It is suggested that the Table be placed in a protective plastic cover or plastic laminate before being affixed to the wall or surface.

Chapter Five
REVIEW EXERCISES

Date _____Name_____

Circle the letters of the terms which most closely approximate the answers. There may be one or more than one correct answer. If you circle D, indicate the other answer or answers, if known.

1. Infection control personnel should be:

   A. younger   B. detail-conscious   C. registered nurses

   D. other_____

2. Infection control education courses should include:

   A. orontology   B. epidemiology   C. paleontology

   D. other_____

3. Office infection control protection begins with:

   A. the first dental visit   B. patient personal care and   C. personnel personal care and
                                    hygiene   hygiene

   D. other_____

4. Dental business office staff may wear:

   A. professional   B. street clothing   C. either gowns or street
      uniforms   clothing

   D. other_____

5. Treatment personnel should wear:

   A. professional   B. street clothing   C. either gowns or street
      uniforms   clothing

   D. other_____

6. Professional uniforms should preferably be:

    A. starched cotton   B. synthetic fiber   C. white

    D. other_____

7. Dentists should wear:

    A. informal dress when   B. fresh professional   C. long sleeved uniforms
       treating children   uniforms

    D. other_____

8. Professional uniforms should be changed:

    A. at least daily   B. at least weekly   C. when dirty

    D. other_____

9. Personnel should not:

    A. wear jewelry   B. wear contacts   C. wear rings

    D. other_____

10. It is all right to have long hair if it is:

    A. clean and carefully   B. covered   C. in a bun
       brushed

    D. other_____

11. All dental staff should wash their hands:

    A. frequently   B. after each patient   C. at least three times each day

    D. other_____

12. Patient evaluation questionnaires are valuable infection control aids because:

    A. patients know their   B. a patient profile is   C. specific questions are asked
       history   provided

    D. other_____

13. Every effort should be made to make infection control:

    A. efficacious   B. practical   C. inexpensive

    D. other_____

14. Routine precautions when treating all patients include:

    A. wearing a mask   B. wearing gloves   C. having patients rinse their
       during treatment   during treatment   mouths

    D. other_____

15. The most important part of washing hands is:

    A. soaping   B. rinsing   C. wash-rinse-wash-rinse-
                                                           wash-rinse

    D. other_____

16. If a hand-activated faucet is used, it should be turned off:

    A. with a paper towel   B. after the patient leaves   C. by the assistant

    D. other_____

17. All soap and lotion dispensers should be:

    A. wall-hung   B. foot or forearm-activated   C. easily disassembled

    D. other_____

18. Cloth towels should:

    A. never be used   B. be changed daily   C. be used only a few times

    D. other_____

19. Eye protection should be:

    A. corrective   B. worn at all times   C. worn at all times when
                                                           treating patients

    D. other_____

20. Face masks are:

A. to be worn at all
times

B. to be worn when treating
patients

C. all effective filters

D. other_____

21. When treating *high risk patients*, dental personnel should:

A. wear gloves at all
times

B. wear gloves during
operative procedures

C. wear finger cots at all times

D. other_____

A. wear disposable
gowns

B. wear gowns one day only

C. wear disposable aprons

D. other_____

A. keep hair in bun

B. wash hair

C. wear hair cover

D. other_____

A. use special waste
container

B. dispose of waste before
treatment

C. dispose of waste after
treatment

D. other_____

A. place contaminated
instruments in
special containers

B. use holding
(pre-cleaning) solution

C. sterilize all surfaces

D. other_____

A. disinfect surfaces
two times after
treatment

B. disinfect surfaces with
special chemical

C. sterilize all surfaces

D. other_____

A. treat dental
equipment routinely

B. treat dental equipment
with special chemical

C. flush water through dental
unit after treatment

D. other_____

NOTE: Answers to review questions appear in the back of this book.

Dental Treatment Areas and the Laboratory

ABSTRACT: Patient treatment areas are exposed to the greatest concentration of potentially pathogenic microorganisms. Microbial control depends, in part, on a cooperative effort of all personnel, closely supervised by the dentist.

Both the private and commercial dental laboratories are often neglected in an infection control program. This neglect can be transformed into a near tragedy, as in the case of the dental laboratory owner who fought hepatitis B for nearly two years.

An effective infection control program requires education, dedication, special attention to detail, continuity, and repetition. Knowledge of infection, epidemiology, microbiology, biochemistry, and certain other sciences is changing, and infection control programs must be constantly evolving to utilize new discoveries. Since dental schools are often slow in assimilating and incorporating change into their teaching programs, dental offices must take the lead in adopting and implementing new aseptic procedures as they are evolved.

Infection control does not produce direct income for the dentist; consequently, the temptation is for the dentist to spend his or her time at the chair and to delegate responsibility for infection control to others. Dentists must provide the continuity in a control program because they are the stabilizing agents in the practice. Other personnel are subject to overly frequent moves and changes. Often, too, they are performing their duties in a "rote" manner, without knowing or particularly caring why they must do what they are doing. This results in a straying from the intended path, unless there is constant, intelligent supervision.

DENTISTS MUST BE INVOLVED IN THE DIRECT IMPLEMENTATION, TRAINING, AND CONTINUING SUPERVISION OF AN EFFECTIVE INFECTION CONTROL PROGRAM.

Patient and personnel protection from infection is possible only when all aspects of dental practice, beginning with the care of the physical facility, are addressed.

Dental treatment areas, sometimes called operatories, examination rooms, x-ray rooms, recovery rooms, and the laboratory offer the highest risk of cross-contamination and infection. It is very important that special care be given to these areas to assure maximum reduction of microbes.

Non-treatment areas also must be considered, but they are of lesser concern than the treatment areas.

Management of Non-Treatment Areas

All non-treatment areas, such as waiting rooms and private and business offices, should be effectively separated from treatment areas as described under planning and office design in a later chapter. Floor coverings, furniture, accessories, and business office equipment should be capable of being easily cleaned, washed, and disinfected whenever necessary.

All non-treatment areas should be dusted and sanitized daily. Special care should be given to areas which may protect microbes, such as coat closets, waste baskets, and lavatories. Carpets should be vacuumed daily, and hard surface floors should be cleaned with a disinfectant detergent at least weekly. All wood surfaces, furniture, arms, and counter tops should be wiped with a cloth or sponge impregnated with a liquid disinfectant.

Air filtration and/or electric sanitizing units are useful in helping reduce microbial count. These devices also reduce office odor, thereby contributing to patient comfort.

Management of Patient Treatment Areas

Following is a suggested schedule for cleaning and disinfecting patient treatment areas.

Monthly

At least once each month, all drawers, cabinets, storage space, and other frequently used areas should be cleaned and disinfected with a long-acting disinfectant. Against certain microbes, some chemicals are effective for long periods of time. Iodophors,[1] for example, are effective for days or even weeks against the hepatitis B virus.

It is not necessary to clean and disinfect seldom used bulk storage areas monthly. Such areas should be treated as necessary, usually twice a year.

Weekly

At least weekly, all hard surfaces, floors, lower part of walls, cabinet fronts, and areas of equipment not disinfected daily should be cleaned and disinfected. A special effort should be made to treat the backs and sides of all portable cabinets and stationary equipment. At times, the temptation exists to clean only those surfaces or parts of equipment easy to reach and only those parts seen by patients. However, microbes usually accumulate in greater numbers in overlooked areas.

Daily

At least daily, high-traffic floors, work surfaces, door knobs, cabinet pulls, and other "touch" surfaces that have not already been disinfected between patients should be wiped with a disinfectant.

Dental units, syringes, hydrocolloid quick-disconnect tubings, ultrasonic scalers, and other water-consuming devices should be flushed with fresh water for as long as possible, at least ten minutes, each morning before use. Water stagnating overnight encourages growth of microbes.

A disinfectant should be circulated through the HVE system after the last use each day. The residual of the disinfectant left in the system will act to help control the growth of microbes when the office is not in use.

Management of the Office Laboratory

The dental laboratory is often an aseptically neglected part of the office, since it is not normally considered a patient treatment area. As a result, the "lab" is potentially a microbiologically dangerous area. Dentures, crowns, bridges, impressions, and other saliva or blood-coated items are carried directly from the patient's mouth to the lab, placed on surfaces, worked on with various instruments and devices, polished by splattering wheels, and then carried back to the patient. Personnel are nearly always exposed to potential infection in the process. If this sounds like an overstatement, consider the case of Mr. Bernard M. Sabatini.

Mr. Sabatini is a certified dental laboratory technician with offices in Hazel Park, Michigan. Sometime in December, 1981, or January, 1982, he picked up a partial denture from the office of one of his dental customers. The partial was in need of repair and had recently been worn by a patient who was later identified as a carrier of hepatitis B.

Mr. Sabatini had accidentally punctured the tip of one of his fingers on a sharp piece of metal the day he handled the partial, and, as a result, conditions were nearly ideal for an infective cross-contamination from the saliva on the partial of the carrier patient to Mr. Sabatini's injured finger. The partial was routinely repaired and returned to the dentist for delivery back to the patient. Since Mr. Sabatini had not been trained in laboratory infection control basics, no microbial reduction procedures were used in his laboratory.

The exposure occurred to Mr. Sabatini in late 1981 or early 1982. He was hospitalized in June, approximately six months later. The presence of a hepatitis B infection was diagnosed and, through a process of elimination related to incubation times, probable etiology of the disease was traced to the infected partial belonging to the hepatitis B carrier. The facts sound like those in a detective story, but it must be realized that disease tracing procedures have been refined to a near science, and it is now possible to identify active carrier infections routinely.

As of this date, Mr. Sabatini is still recovering from the effects of the infection and he has only recently returned to work. Inasmuch as a significant number of hepatitis patients die each year, he is fortunate to have survived. As might be expected, Mr. Sabatini has become an active advocate of infection control in the dental laboratory. He is writing articles[2] and lecturing on his experience in an effort to help save others from the same problems.

Can this same experience happen in the private dental laboratory? Of course, since statistically five to twenty-five percent of persons involved in dental procedures in the United States are exposed to hepatitis B in the conduct of their profession or business. Laboratory technicians are not exceptions, and these statistics are for hepatitis only. Emerging diseases such as herpes II and AIDS must also be considered risks with possible transmission to and from dental laboratories.

Handling Prostheses

Before working on a prosthesis in the laboratory or before sending a prosthesis to a commercial laboratory, the assistant or technician should thoroughly clean the device with a dilute disinfectant detergent, such as iodophor and water or phenolic compound and water. If the device is non-metal, it should be immersed in an EPA registered iodophor hard surface disinfectant, phenolic compound, or glutaraldehyde.

A 1984 study from Indiana University School of Dentistry[3] has shown "that dental impression materials can easily become contaminated with patients' blood and saliva during the impression process." Anyone handling such impressions is subject to cross-contamination.

Microorganisms have been shown to be transferred from impressions into the stone casts made from such impressions. A 1983 study from the University of Southern California, School of Dentistry, stated, "The recovery of microorganisms from the stone cast shows that dental casts may be a medium of cross-contamination between patients and dental personnel. Laboratory personnel handling casts from patients with known communicable diseases (especially viral hepatitis) should take precautions to prevent personal infection and possible disease transmission to other dental patients and personnel. When such casts are handled, gloves should be used and materials sterilized or discarded."[4]

The process of spreading potential infection through the laboratory is very real.

All impressions should be rinsed under gently running water to mechanically remove debris, blood, and saliva. Whenever possible, impressions should be soaked in diluted iodophor or other EPA disinfectant solution for at least ten minutes. Of course, care should be exercised not to distort the impression.

Much investigation remains to be done on the effects of treatment of impressions with disinfectant; however, the same Indiana study previously cited showed that iodophor, one glutaraldehyde and an iodophor/alcohol mixture had no dimensional effect on alginate impressions. Diluted bleach showed slightly more dimensional change. On a basis of this work, dilute EPA registered hard surface iodophor disinfectant is the material of choice for disinfecting impressions. Household bleach should be used when iodophor is not available. Dental gypsum products, such as casts and jaw relation records, should never be scrubbed or allowed to soak in anything other than saturated slurry water.

Grinding and Polishing

A liquid disinfectant dilution, such as iodophor or hypochlorite, should be used as the mixing medium for pumice. Adding three parts of green soap in the disinfectant solution will keep pumice suspended.[5] Two pumice pans should be used. One pan should be saved for new prostheses, and the pumice should be changed daily. A second pan should be used for prostheses which have been in the mouth, and the pumice should be changed after each patient. To save time, one may mix pumice weekly and package it in small containers. It is quick and simple to wash out the old pumice and add the new pre-packaged pumice. Of course, it takes a little effort . . . but it is much less effort than fighting hepatitis as Mr. Sabatini had to do.

Laboratory attachments, such as burs and rag wheels, should be kept separate for new prostheses and for prostheses that have been in the mouth. Laboratory attachments used on new prostheses should be sterilized daily, and attachments used on prostheses that have been in the

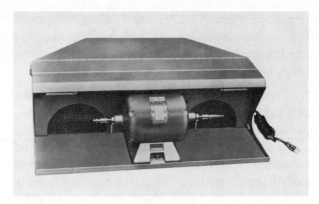

FIGURE 19
Lab filtering evacuator.

mouth should be sterilized after each use. Rag wheels should be washed and sterilized in an autoclave. Since bristle brushes may be damaged in a heat sterilization system, such brushes should be rinsed well and placed in undiluted glutaraldehyde for the manufacturer's recommended sterilization time. The brushes must then be rinsed with sterile water before use. After each use, adjusting burs and stones should be ultrasonically cleaned and sterilized in a chemical vapor sterilizer. After being polished, new or repaired prostheses should be cleaned as described above and rinsed before delivery to the patient.

Precautions

To prevent contaminated material from being recirculated in the laboratory or carried to patient areas, dental personnel should make sure that all lathes, grinders, and lab handpieces are connected to or used near a dust-chip evacuation system containing a filter. (See Figure 19.)

In addition to the precautions for the handling of prostheses, there are many other precautions that must be observed in the laboratory.

Before working in the laboratory, staff should carefully wash their hands, particularly if transferring items and/or equipment to and from the treatment area and the laboratory.

Certain treatment procedures require the use of equipment and supplies often kept in the laboratory. This is especially true in prosthodontic[6] and crown and bridge treatment. All equipment and supplies transferred between the two areas must be sterilized or disinfected before and after use on a patient.

All consumables used in or near the patient's mouth, such as impression materials, bite registrations, or wax and similar substances, should be disposable and discarded after a single use. Similarly, all carriers for disposable materials used in the mouth, such as impression trays and bite registration frames, should be disposed of or cleaned and sterilized after each use.

After patient treatment is completed, disposable items should be discarded. Instruments and smaller equipment should be processed in the instrument recirculation center, and larger equipment should be thoroughly disinfected before being returned to the laboratory.

Some routine laboratory procedures, such as the construction of crowns, bridges, partials and full dentures, do not involve direct patient treatment after the casts have been prepared. Infectious exposure to staff is substantially reduced during such non-patient laboratory work. Nevertheless, there is always danger of contamination of laboratory instruments, surfaces, and equipment by airborne or staff-borne pathogens. It is necessary to frequently disinfect all laboratory work surfaces and exposed equipment, such as lathes, vibrators, handpieces, ovens, casting machines, and similar items, preferably daily in areas of high usage. Additionally, frequently used instruments, such as spatulas, saws, wax carvers, and similar items should be sterilized daily. Of course, sterilization should be preceded by gross removal of all wax, plaster, rubber or silicone materials, followed by a final ultrasonic cleaning.

Frequently used drawers, containers, and case identification boxes should be cleaned and disinfected periodically. Case identification boxes should be treated after completion of each case.

All personnel working in the laboratory should exercise careful personal hygiene. Clothing should be clean and should be changed as necessary. Technicians should wear fresh uniforms whenever assisting the dentist in the operatory. When using laboratory equipment, for example

when adjusting and polishing a denture, the staff assisting with patient treatment should wear disposable aprons to protect clean professional uniforms.

Finally, and very significantly, private offices should attempt to protect commercial laboratory personnel from infection when sending impressions, casts, broken prostheses, or other devices or materials to commercial laboratories for processing. EACH ITEM SHOULD BE CLEANED OF BLOOD AND SALIVA AND SHOULD BE WASHED AND/OR DISINFECTED AS PREVIOUSLY DESCRIBED. The items should be sealed in plastic bags containing disinfectant, unless the moist chemical will harm the item. If the prosthesis is from a high risk patient, the plastic bag or shipping container should be clearly marked with an external warning label such as: *"Special handling required. Contents are biologically high risk."* This pre-treatment and warning notification may prove to be a valuable aid in reducing cross-contamination to laboratory technicians.

Office should also request that all cases are disinfected by the laboratory before return to the office.

Management of the Commercial Laboratory

The commercial laboratory is confronted with infection control problems somewhat different from those found in the dental office laboratory. Cases are sent to the laboratory from diverse types of practices; therefore, commercial laboratory personnel have little knowledge of or control over procedures or precautions practiced by any dentist in his or her office. It is very important that the commercial laboratory observe certain infection control precautions in addition to those exercised by the dental offices.

Following is a list of those precautions which should be observed.

79

Precautions

1. All personnel handling prostheses, models, impressions, or other items sent by dental offices should consider being vaccinated against hepatitis B and other infectious diseases.

2. Personnel opening packages from dental offices should wear utility gloves and should be especially careful with packages labeled for special handling.

3. All wrapping and packaging materials, which have been in contact with prostheses, models, impressions, or other items that have been in a patient's mouth, should be discarded and not re-used.

   Hands should be washed as described previously immediately after handling potentially contaminated cases.

4. The receiving and shipping bench(es) should be disinfected at least daily, and always after each case is received, to prevent contamination of outgoing cases.

   If sodium hypochlorite (household bleach) is used as a disinfectant, care should be exercised to avoid damaging or injuring clothing, skin, or eyes. Iodophor solution is safer to use and is also inexpensive.

   Because of the potentially corrosive effect hypochlorite may have on metals in laboratories, iodophors are the disinfectants of choice.

5. All appliances, impressions, or other oral items received from customer dental offices should be disinfected for ten minutes before being routed to laboratory departments. Care should be exercised not to damage the case.

6. Disinfecting solutions should be changed frequently, preferably daily in areas of heavy usage.

7. Hands should be washed frequently with an antibacterial soap, and hands should always be washed when changing cases.

8. Work gowns should be changed frequently, preferably daily.

9. Case work containers, sometimes called pans or trays, should be disinfected (sterilized if possible) each time a case is completed.

10. Ultrasonic cleaning solution should be changed frequently, preferably daily in areas of heavy usage, and the cleaner should be used only with the lid securely in place to prevent solution aerosol.

11. Disinfectant solution should be mixed with pumice and three parts green soap for suspension of the solution. Pumice used on repairs should be changed after each case, and pumice used on new cases should be changed frequently, preferably daily in areas of heavy usage.

12. Work benches should be disinfected at least daily.

13. Sinks and wash areas should be cleaned and disinfected daily.

14. Personnel should not eat at their work stations.

15. Conscientious housekeeping procedures should be observed in all non-work areas.

16. Be careful not to mix household bleach with other solutions containing alcohol or ammonia.

17. Encourage the expanded use of patient medical history in the dental office, then relayed to the laboratory with the prescription. The use of case warning labels on the outside of packages to indicate special precautions to be observed before opening the package should be requested of each dental customer.

18. Laboratory personnel seeing patients for the purpose of shade verification for dentures or bridgework must be sure the shade room is clean and properly disinfected before and after the patient leaves the laboratory. Shade buttons or other items that have been in the patient's mouth, or anything touched with fingers that have been in the patient's mouth, must be disinfected immediately. Disposable rubber gloves, a mask, and eye protection should be worn if the patient is coughing or if the patient has a history of any contagious disease.

80

TABLE 9
Laboratory Receiving and Polishing, Cleaning and Disinfecting Procedures
Minimal Program

Receiving Cases
1. Wear latex utility gloves when opening packages.
2. Discard all disposable packing materials. Disinfect all returnable containers.
3. Rinse all impressions, dentures, try-ins, repairs, etc., under running water. Take care not to splash.
4. Soak or spray all items with DILUTE iodophor, or other EPA-registered disinfectant.
5. Route case to appropriate department.
6. After work is completed, treat finished case again with iodophor or other EPA-registered disinfectant before returning to customer.
7. Clean and disinfect all work stations and receiving-shipping bench between each case.
Grinding and Polishing
8. Replace pumice at least daily and mix with iodophor or other EPA disinfectant. Use disposable plastic liner.
9. Soak brushes, rag wheels, etc., overnight in glutaraldehyde, iodophor, or other EPA disinfectant.

The Table on the reverse of this page is designed to be placed on the wall or other surface as a constant reminder of information which might be otherwise forgotten

It is suggested that the Table be placed in a protective plastic cover or plastic laminate before being affixed to the wall or surface.

References and Suggested Readings

1. Centers for Disease Control, U.S. Department of Health, Education and Welfare. "Hepatitis Control Measures for Hepatitis B in Dialysis Centers," Nov 1977, Viral Hepatitis Investigation Control Series.

2. Sabatini, B.M. "Don't Let It Happen To You," Oct, 1982, Ntl Assoc of Dent Lab, 19.

3. Setcos, *et al.* "The Effect of Disinfection Procedures on An Alginate Impression Material," Apr, 1984, Dent Asep Rev, 1.

4. Leung, R., Schonfeld, S. "Gympsum Casts As A Potential Source of Microbial Cross-contamination," Feb, 1983, Jnl of Pros Dent, 210.

5. Matis, Young, *et al.* "Infection Control in Air Force Dental Clinics," Dec, 1980, Aeromed Rev, USAF Schl of Aerosp Med, Brooks AF Base, Texas.

6. Whitacre, R. and Stern, M. "Avoiding Cross-contamination in Prosthetics," Aug, 1981, The Jnl of Prost Dent, 46:2, Aug, 1981, 120-122.

Chapter Six
REVIEW EXERCISES

Date _____ Name_____

Circle the letters of the terms which most closely approximate the answers. There may be one or more than one correct answer. If you circle D, indicate the other answer or answers, if known.

1. All non-treatment areas should be:

   A. sanitized daily   B. disinfected daily   C. cleaned daily

   D. other_____

2. When cleaning and disinfecting treatment areas, personnel should:

   A. disinfect frequently used cabinets weekly   B. disinfect frequently used cabinets monthly   C. disinfect frequently used cabinets twice a year

   D. other_____

3. When cleaning and disinfecting treatment areas, personnel should:

   A. disinfect hard surfaces and floors weekly   B. disinfect front of cabinets only   C. sanitize handles of cabinet

   D. other_____

4. When cleaning and disinfecting treatment areas, personnel should:

   A. disinfect "touch" surfaces daily   B. disinfect "touch" surfaces between patients   C. disinfect HVE system each day

   D. other_____

5. When cleaning and disinfecting treatment areas, personnel should:

   A. flush dental units each morning   B. flush ultrasonic scalers each morning   C. flush hydrocolloid quick-disconnect tubings each morning

   D. other_____

6. When handling dental prostheses, office and commercial laboratory personnel should:

A. use a disinfectant

B. put metal in sodium hypochlorite

C. rinse impressions under water

D. other_____

7. When grinding and polishing prostheses, busy office and commercial laboratory personnel should:

A. change pumice at least monthly

B. change pumice at least daily

C. change pumice at least weekly

D. other_____

8. When grinding and polishing prostheses, office and commercial laboratory personnel should:

A. wear safety glasses

B. wear heavy rubber gloves

C. use lathe eye shields

D. other_____

9. Rag wheels used on new prostheses should be:

A. disinfected daily

B. sterilized weekly

C. sterilized monthly

D. other_____

10. Commercial laboratory personnel should:

A. wear gloves when opening incoming packages

B. observe warning labels

C. wear aprons

D. other_____

11. Commercial laboratory personnel should disinfect shipping and receiving bench:

A. at least daily

B. at least weekly

C. after every hazardous container is received

D. other_____

12. Commercial laboratory work containers should be:

A. disinfected daily

B. sterilized

C. disinfected or sterilized each time case is changed

D. other_____

NOTE: Answers to the review questions appear in the back of this book.

Preparing To Receive Patients

ABSTRACT: Since much of the office cannot be sterilized, cleaning and disinfection are very important. Disinfectants are often misunderstood and mis-used.

An effective program of disinfection must also include use of microbial barriers and one-use disposables.

It is important to recognize that patients have become much more aware of infection control protection offered by professional offices. Because of the media attention given to the AIDS threat, many patients have been "educated" that dental practitioners and their staffs should be observing at least SIX BASIC INFECTION CONTROL PROCEDURES. These six procedures are emphasized by the CDC, ADA, and many infection control experts. Emphasis is placed on the following:

1) All treatment personnel should wear protective eyewear during treatment procedures.

2) All treatment personnel should wear protective masks during treatment procedures.

3) All treatment personnel should wear latex examination gloves during treatment procedures.

4) All "critical" instruments and items used in or near the mouth should be sterilized in a heat or heat-pressure sterilizer, not a liquid.

5) All "touch and splash" surfaces should be carefully disinfected with an intermediate or higher EPA/ADA disinfectant.

6) Potentially contaminated waste should be disposed of very carefully.

Preparation of the treatment area for the next patient is very "visible" to many aware patients.

Before a patient is received, the treatment room should be completely cleaned, disinfected, and prepared. Because any mistake may result in cross-contamination, thoroughness is a necessity.

The procedures are the same whether personnel are preparing to treat the first patient in the day or whether they are preparing the treatment room between patients. Some offices prepare a treatment area at the end of the day in preparation for the first patient the next morning. It is much better to prepare the treatment area each time just before the patient is presented for treatment because there is little control over happenings after the office has been closed. Janitorial services often create contaminated splashes, or they wipe surfaces with contaminated cloths. Additionally, personnel are often in

87

a hurry to get home, and late afternoon procedures may be rushed.

Preparation of a treatment area to receive a patient should consist of cleaning and disinfecting various surfaces and equipment; placing disposable items (saliva ejectors, HVE tips, etc.) on equipment; and covering as many surfaces, handles, and other "touch areas" as possible with a disposable barrier.

Instrument Recirculation and Cleaning

Before considering disinfectant products and techniques, it is very important to consider cleaning. ALL DISINFECTING AND STERILIZING PROCEDURES ARE 2-STEP PROCEDURES. FIRST CLEAN, THEN DISINFECT OR STERILIZE. The success of either procedure depends on efficiently completing the cleaning procedure first.

A study by the Centers for Disease Control of the inactivation of hepatitis B virus by disinfectants pointed out:

THE MOST IMPORTANT STEP IN ANY DISINFECTING [AND STERILIZING] PROTOCOL IS ADEQUATE PRECLEANING OF SURFACES BEFORE CONDUCTING THE ACTUAL DISINFECTING [AND STERILIZING] STEP.[1]

Organic debris left on surfaces not only may interfere with the action of the disinfectant, but also may contain massive numbers of microorganisms. A simple scrubbing, followed by a water rinse of the soiled surface, will enhance the disinfecting action substantially. Personnel must observe procedures which clean the surfaces and which do not just spread the contaminants to other surfaces, as is often done when personnel attempt to conserve the use of sponges or toweling and cleaning and disinfecting agents. Contaminated "wipe" materials should be properly discarded after each use. Of course, personnel should always use heavy latex utility rubber gloves during the cleaning and disinfecting procedures. After the cleaning is completed, all surfaces should be disinfected.

SURFACE DISINFECTION SHOULD ALWAYS INCLUDE TWO STEPS—CLEANING AND THEN DISINFECTING.

RECIRCULATION INSTRUCTIONS

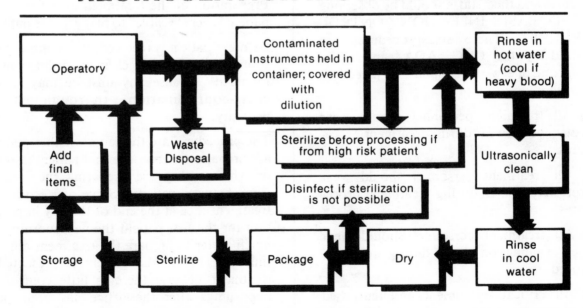

FIGURE 20
Recirculation procedures.

Cleaning of instruments and items to be disinfected or sterilized is very important. A repetitious method of "instrument recirculation" assures the most effective cleaning of contaminated items. Additionally, such method offers the greatest degree of protection to dental personnel by minimizing handling and hand-scrubbing of instruments. Figure 20 on the previous page outlines the most efficient recirculation of instruments and items. IT IS VERY IMPORTANT TO COMPLETE EACH STEP AS SUMMARIZED BELOW. ELIMINATING OR COMPROMISING STEPS MAY DEFEAT EFFECTIVE STERILIZATION OR DISINFECTION AND MAY EXPOSE PERSONNEL TO NEEDLESS CROSS-CONTAMINATION.

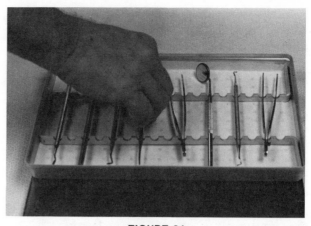

FIGURE 21
Unpackaged instruments in freshly lined tray, spread apart for minimum contamination use.

Steps in instrument recirculation, as outlined in Figure 20, are as follows:

1. Holding (pre-cleaning) provides the earliest possible microbial reduction and prevents drying of blood, serum, saliva, and debris on instruments. The holding procedure is more fully described later in this chapter.

2. Rinsing of contaminated instruments in hot water (cool if blood is present, then followed by hot) assures most efficient ultrasonic cleaning.

3. Ultrasonic cleaning is the most efficient method of removal of blood, serum, saliva, and debris.[2] Additionally, ultrasonic cleaning minimizes handling of instruments by personnel, thereby minimizing possible exposure to contaminants through finger cuts and nicks. Of course, latex utility gloves should always be worn by clean-up and treatment personnel when handling contaminated instruments after patient treatment has been completed.

4. Following ultrasonic cleaning, solution and soap should be rinsed from instruments and items to assure that the items are clean before sterilization or disinfection. Soap may bake on instruments in certain sterilizers.

5. Instruments and items should be dried by placing on a PAPER towel and patting with another PAPER towel. Used towels should be discarded after each use. CLOTH TOWELS SHOULD NOT BE RE-USED FOR DRYING BECAUSE OF GROWTH OF ORGANISMS IN MOIST TOWELING.

6. Instruments should be pre-packaged wherever possible before sterilization and then stored following sterilization. If instruments are to be re-used immediately following sterilization, the pre-packaging step may be eliminated AS LONG AS INSTRUMENTS ARE NOT PLACED IN POTENTIALLY CONTAMINATED DRAWERS BETWEEN USERS. If instruments are to be stored unpackaged for reasonably immediate use, Figure 21 illustrates a method of storing in an open tray which minimizes contamination by retrieving and replacing instruments between usage. IT IS VERY IMPORTANT IN OPEN STORAGE TO CLEAN AND DISINFECT ALL STORAGE TRAYS AT LEAST DAILY. A LINER SHOULD BE PLACED IN THE BOTTOM OF THE TRAY OR BETWEEN THE TRAY AND THE INSTRUMENTS AND THE LINER DISCARDED DAILY IF PRACTICAL. USE FOR MORE THAN SEVERAL DAYS SHOULD BE DISCOURAGED.

7. All items which can be sterilized without damage in a sterilizer should be sterilized. Sterilization is more completely described in a later chapter.

8. If sterilization is not possible, items should be disinfected in an efficacious and properly registered disinfectant. IN THE TREATMENT OF RISK AND HIGH RISK PATIENTS, DISINFECTION SHOULD NEVER BE USED IN PLACE OF STERILIZATION WHEN STERILIZATION IS POSSIBLE.

9. All sterilized packaged items should be stored out of traffic to prevent possible recontamination through the packaging. It is preferable to not store sterilized materials in the treatment area. Closed cabinets and seldom-used drawers offer reasonable protection from recontamination during storage.

A method of holding (pre-cleaning) of soiled instruments in the treatment area is very important if soiled instruments cannot be cleaned within a few minutes after use. Because many instruments remain on the bracket table for minutes to hours, pre-cleaning is an important adjunct to instrument recirculation.[3] Holding (pre-cleaning) is a procedure which has been used in medicine for years. Holding is a term which has been misused in some disciplines to indicate placing instruments in a solution AFTER sterilization. Of course, such treatment should not be used.

Holding, properly defined, is the process of placing used and/or soiled instruments and other items in a solution immediately after use (preferably chairside during treatment) and BEFORE CLEANING AND STERILIZATION OR DISINFECTION. Figures 22-29 on the following pages illustrate the steps of a holding (and ultrasonic cleaning) procedure.

Holding (pre-cleaning) soiled instruments provides the following advantages:

1. Prevents bioburden and debris from drying on instruments and thereby makes cleaning easier and safer.

2. Minimizes hand-scrubbing with the potential for staff infection from cuts on the hands.

3. Begins microbial kill at chairside (the earliest possible time).

4. Prevents airborne transmission of dried microorganisms.

5. Keeps patients from looking at bloody and soiled instruments.

Holding (pre-cleaning) is relatively new to dentistry, and should be considered as an advancement of the state-of-the-art of microbial control and patient and staff protection.

If instruments are not held in a holding solution at chairside, they should be placed in a holding solution immediately after patient treatment is completed and the patient has been dismissed. However, time has elapsed and the benefits of chairside holding are lost.

The phenolic compounds are excellent holding agents, either in the disinfecting dilution (1:32) or the sanitizing dilution (1:128).

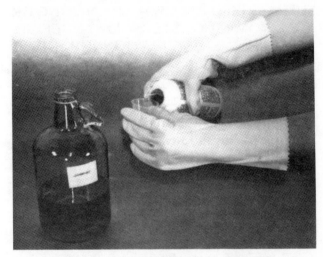

FIGURE 22
Mixing holding (pre-cleaning) solution.

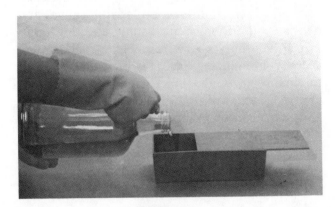

FIGURE 23
Placing holding solution in tray.

CLEANING IS VERY IMPORTANT TO EFFICACIOUS INSTRUMENT RECIRCULATION, INCLUDING DISINFECTION AND STERILIZATION.

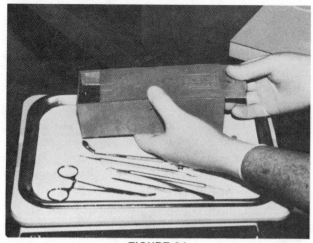

FIGURE 24
Placing tray on (or near) bracket table.

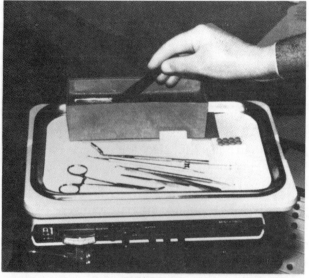

FIGURE 25
Placing instrument into holding solution after final use.

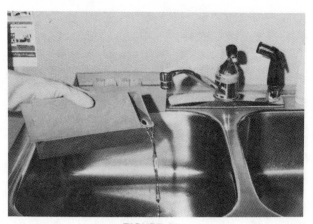

FIGURE 26
Pouring solution down drain after holding and pre-cleaning instruments.

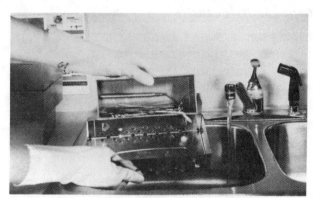

FIGURE 27
"Rolling" instruments into ultrasonic tray.

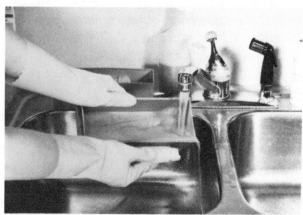

FIGURE 28
Cleaning tray with soap and copious water after use.

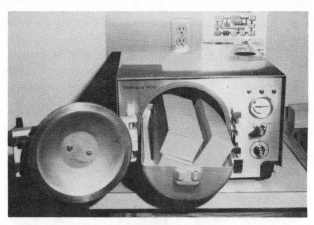

FIGURE 29
Sterilizing trays in autoclave or Chemiclave.

Categories of Liquid Sterilants and Disinfectants

Liquid sterilants and disinfectants may be classified into at least four broad categories: (1) surface disinfectants, (2) immersion (instrument) sterilants, (3) immersion disinfectants, and (4) hand antimicrobials. Each category is distinguished by different needs, and care should be exercised to separate the categories; otherwise confusion may result.

Surface disinfection is the treatment of cabinets, bracket tables, chairs, units, lights, x-rays and similar surfaces where the items are too large to be immersed in the disinfecting chemical. Immersion disinfection (sometimes called instrument disinfection or incorrectly "cold sterilization") is the immersion of instruments, plastics, and other smaller items in a liquid disinfectant contained in a disinfecting tray, historically called a "cold sterilizing" tray. Immersion sterilization is the use of an EPA registered agent that has the capability of killing all living microorganisms and infective agents in the recommended immersion time. Hand antimicrobial treatment is the specific art of washing or otherwise treating hands with a chemical soap or lotion which results in a substantial reduction in the number of hand microbes.

Much of the confusion in dentistry concerning disinfectants is a result of misunderstanding of these three broad disinfectant categories. In the search for simplicity and economy, dental personnel often attempt to use a single chemical to satisfy diverse office needs. Each surface, immersion or hand antimicrobial has certain limitations and should be used accordingly.

Another area of confusion is comprehending shelf-life, use-life, and re-use life. Shelf-life is time that a product remains effective WHEN STORED in the original undiluted and/or unmixed form. For example, certain glutaraldehydes must be mixed with an activator, and this category of product has a shelf-life of only several weeks after mixing. Some products do not require mixing and have an extended shelf-life, which, in this case, is also the use-life. Shelf-life, while important, is less important than use-life and re-use life.

Use-life is the effective life after dilution and/or mixing BUT WITHOUT BEING USED. Re-use life is the time a product is effective IN ACTUAL USE. Re-use life may vary greatly depending upon the number of patients treated; the amount of bio-burden and water introduced into the disinfectant; whether the container is kept closed to prevent oxidation; the amount of ultrasonic cleaning solution remaining on items placed in the solution; and a number of other variables. While testing protocols exist for projecting re-use life, they are designed to simulate practical use conditions and, therefore, such tests are, at best, somewhat subjective.

The only way to assure an efficacious re-use life is to change solutions frequently, daily or more often as needed. Highly disciplined offices, where use of solutions is minimal, may be able to extend re-use life safely; but use of any product should never exceed the manufacturer's EPA registered product claim as printed on the label.

If the EPA registered label of a product does not specify a re-use claim and instructions, products must be discarded daily.

Regulatory Compliance

In addition to use considerations, there are regulatory or compliance and acceptance standards which must be considered when selecting sterilizing or disinfecting chemicals. The laws and guidelines governing federal registration of all chemicals for which disinfecting and sterilizing claims are made is discussed more completely in a later chapter. In summary, certain products must be registered with the Environmental Protection Agency (EPA) if the products are to be used on inanimate surfaces, instruments, or objects. The Federal Drug Administration (FDA) administers registration of chemicals to be used on or in the human body. Additionally, the American Dental Association (ADA) includes most disinfecting and sterilizing agents or processes in the ADA Acceptance Program, thereby corroborating that the products function as claimed under the EPA registration.

Knowledge of these regulatory and acceptance programs is necessary for intelligent product evaluation. Additionally, malpractice considerations are rapidly making a knowledge of Federal law mandatory as discussed in Chapter 8. Professionals treating patients without proper knowledge of the correct use of disinfectants may be suspected of compromising patient treatment.

On a more positive side, knowledge of regulatory laws and acceptance programs allows enlightened personnel to make more considered judgments of products and to determine the correct use thereof.

Selection of Specific Chemicals

For many years in dentistry, disinfection meant the use of one or more quaternary ammonium compounds (benzalkonium chloride, dibenzalkonium chloride, cetyldimethylethylammonium bromide, cetylpyridinium chloride, and alkyldimethylbenzylammonium chloride) in low concentrations or alcohol on instruments and handpieces. A number of researchers[4] and agencies, such as the Centers for Disease Control (CDC) and the ADA, have publicized the limitations of "quats" and alcohol.[5] Recent studies[6] [7] have shown that these same two chemicals are still used in 50%-70% of U.S. dental offices. And yet, the ADA Council on Dental Therapeutics published a report in 1978[8] titled "Quaternary Ammonium Not Acceptable for Use in Dental Offices." Such warnings found limited acceptance until viral hepatitis was shown to be a potentially serious problem in dental offices and laboratories.[9] [10] More recently, concerns for the transmission of herpes simplex I[11] [12] and the possible transmission of herpes II (genital type) and AIDS[13] [14] to dental personnel, and remotely to patients, has catalyzed interest in the subject.

With these increased concerns has also come an interest in infection control by a number of researchers, clinicians and commercial groups. The dissemination of new and old information has been rapid, and even the most serious students of the subject have difficulty in filtering fact from fiction.

As a point of reference for comparing disinfectants, Table 10 on the following page lists the properties of an ideal disinfectant.

The generic categories of chemical sterilants/disinfectants acceptable and efficacious for practical use in dentistry include glutaraldehydes, iodophors, a phenolic compound, and chlorine dioxide. Certain other products, for example peroxide, may eventually prove acceptable; however, such products need more diverse office use before their practical value to dentistry can be assessed.

Other products have been considered for use in dentistry, for example sodium hypochlorite, but have been found to be deficient for practical use. Sodium hypochlorite (household bleach) bleaches clothing, cloth, and painted walls, damages certain kinds of metal, particularly carbon steel and aluminum, and has an undesirable odor. Sodium hypochlorite is also not EPA registered for use as a dental disinfectant at this writing.

Quaternary Ammonium Compounds

Quaternary ammonium compounds and alcohol have not been recommended for use in dentistry since much of the original work in the mid-seventies. "Quats" are irregularly virucidal, do not kill the tubercle bacillus, are inactivated by soap, and are easily neutralized by bioburden, such as blood, serum and saliva. Quats should not be used for disinfection in the dental office.

TABLE 10
Properties of An Ideal Disinfectant

1. **Broad Spectrum:**
   - Should always have the widest possible antimicrobial spectrum.

2. **Fast Acting:**
   - Should always have a rapidly lethal action on all vegetative forms and spores of bacteria and fungi, protozoa and viruses.

3. **Not Affected by Physical Factors:**
   - Active in the presence of organic matter such as blood, sputum and feces.
   - Should be compatible with soaps, detergents and other chemicals encountered in use.

4. **Not Toxic**

5. **Surface Compatibility:**
   - Should not corrode instruments and other metallic surfaces.
   - Should not cause the disintegration of cloth, rubber, plastics, or other materials.

6. **Residual Effect on Treated Surfaces**

7. **Easy To Use**

8. **Odorless:**
   - An inoffensive odor would facilitate its routine use.

9. **Economical:**
   - Cost should not be prohibitively high.

10. **Registered with the EPA and Accepted by the ADA**

Adapted from: Molinari, J.A.; Campbell, M.D.; and York, J.: "Minimizing Potential Infections in Dental Practice." J. Michigan Dent Assoc 64:411-416 (1982).

Alcohols

Alcohol has been studied by a number of researchers for years and has been found to be irregularly virucidal against certain of the more resistant viruses. Alcohol is not sporicidal, evaporates too rapidly, and does not allow sufficient time to assure dependably continuous action.

Alcohol does not contain soap or surfactants which assist in cleaning. Cleaning agents are important to aid in the preparation of surfaces or items for disinfection or sterilization.

Alcohol has NOT been recommended by researchers for a number of years, and the CDC and the ADA have both published guidelines specifically stating that alcohol should not be used. In case of an infection control legal action against an office using alcohol, it may be difficult to justify use of a product on which substantial negative information has been published. Representative excerpts concerning alcohol are as follows:

> . . . *alcohol dries too quickly to assure effectiveness against all dried viruses in saliva or blood of unrecognized carriers, although it is said to kill HBV in 2 minutes. Alcohol is not licensed [registered] as a disinfectant.* [15]

> *Alcohols have been shown to be excellent antiseptics for epidermis and hands [if used for 30 seconds or longer], but their use for disinfection of dental instruments is highly discouraged, both because of lack of evidence they can destroy hepatitis viruses and because of their inability to penetrate organic and cellular material on instruments. Furthermore, rapid evaporation limits surface area.* [16]

Finally, alcohol is not registered with the EPA as a surface disinfectant as is required under the FIFR Act. Use of a non-registered product poses a potential problem of efficacy and legality.

Glutaraldehydes

Compounds of two percent glutaraldehydes are either sterilants or disinfectants, depending on dilution and exposure time. In order to sterilize, glutaraldehydes must be used full strength for 6¾ hours for one product and ten hours for all others at room temperature, or one to four hours at elevated or potentiated temperatures. [17] Some researchers have expressed reservations about heating glutaraldehyde, except in a closed system, because of the potentially increased toxicity of the vapors at elevated temperatures. It is prudent to review such studies before adopting the heat potentiated systems. Glutaraldehydes biodegrade slowly.

Glutaraldehydes are effective disinfectants when used for shorter periods of time, varying from 10 to 90 minutes. [18] Recent testing protocols have shown that up to 90 minutes' exposure time is required for destruction of large numbers of *Mycobacterium tuberculosis.* [19]

From a practical standpoint, because it is nearly impossible to know when a specific microbe is present, the disinfection time of any chemical should always be the longest of the recommended exposure times.

Manufacturers of glutaraldehydes are being asked to furnish the EPA with new product efficacy data to prove both shelf-life and re-use life claims, if manufacturers wish a re-use claim. Some glutaraldehyde manufacturers now provide chemical tests for indicating when the concentration of the chemical drops below the one percent critical level. Use of such tests partially solves the re-use life problem, although the tests have not been perfected.

Because all properly EPA registered glutaraldehydes are registered for use only as immersion sterilants or disinfectants, *they should not be used for surface disinfection.* [20] Additionally, evaporation of glutaraldehydes from large environmental surfaces may present a vapor toxicity problem.

Iodophors

Iodophors are complexes of iodine in a slow

release mechanism usually containing a cleaning agent. There are two categories of iodophors — skin antimicrobials or sanitizers (often called surgical scrubs) and hard surface iodophors. Both categories release iodine in the same manner, but action on animate or inanimate surfaces is different. Iodophors release a predictable low percentage of the free iodine molecule, depending on the type and concentration of the compound. Accordingly, iodophors discolor surfaces substantially less than does free iodine. This is particularly true of the hard surface iodophors, which do not discolor hard surfaces such as formica. Iodophors are more effective in an optimum dilution than in a higher concentrate,[21] and they should be used in strict accordance with manufacturer's instructions.

Iodophors are also relatively non-toxic, and as a result, they are used extensively in the dairy, ice cream, and beverage industries for sanitizing or disinfecting equipment and cow teats before milking. Because iodine, the basic ingredient of iodophors, is a naturally occurring substance, iodophors are rapidly biodegradable.

Iodophors also provide efficacious disinfection of hard surfaces, such as cabinet tops, light handles, x-ray heads and arms, and similar objects. EPA registered hard surface iodophors should be mixed 213 parts soft or distilled water to one part iodophor concentrate and should be used generously on surfaces for at least ten minutes. Pre-cleaning is very important in any disinfecting treatment,[22] and iodophors contain a soap additive which aids in the cleaning process. HOWEVER, PARTICULARLY SOILED OR CONTAMINATED AREAS SHOULD BE CLEANED AND TREATED A SECOND TIME WITH FRESH IODOPHOR TO ASSURE MAXIMUM DISINFECTION. Iodophor should be disposed of whenever the color changes substantially, to very light yellow or clear, thereby indicating that the free and available iodine is exhausted.

While properly EPA registered iodophors may be used for both surfaces and instruments, certain metals, most particularly carbon steel and aluminum, will be discolored and/or damaged if left too long in the solution. Because such deleterious effect is cumulative,[23] it is particularly important with iodophors to remove instruments immediately after the manufacturer's specified disinfecting time.

Iodophors also are effective hand detergents, but they have short-term residual action after washing,[24] and therefore, they are less desirable for dentistry than other hand-treatment chemicals which offer continuing antimicrobial action on hands for hours after use.[25] Parachlorometaxylenol (PCMX) and chlorhexidine gluconate provide longer residual action when incorporated into hand soaps.

Phenolics

Phenols were not recommended for use in dentistry for some years.[26] However, a new generation of this category of disinfectant is evolving. A compound of synthetic phenolics has recently been studied by researchers and the ADA and has been shown to be efficacious for disinfection of instruments and items which can be immersed in the dilute compound for 10-20 minutes.[27] The new phenolic products have several advantages in that they effectively destroy a broad spectrum of microbes (a deficiency of simple phenol), and they are relatively inexpensive in the recommended 1:32 dilution with water. There are no negative handling characteristics or objectionable odors. While historical phenols were often destructive to certain instruments, the new phenolic compounds contain chemicals which preclude instrument damage for a number of hours.[28]

Additionally, the action of the new phenolic compounds is synergistic rather than additive.[29] The synthetic phenolic compounds may also be diluted up to 1:128 to serve as a sanitizing (not disinfecting) holding solution. Placing instruments in a holding solution, described more fully later in this chapter, immediately after use assures more effective pre-cleaning by preventing the drying of blood, serum, or other debris on such instruments. Holding also minimizes environmental contamination by airborne microbes.

As with all disinfectants, it is highly desirable to discard solutions daily to assure maximal efficaciousness.

Chlorine Dioxides

A new sterilant/disinfectant, chlorine dioxide, has recently been introduced into use in dentistry. While the product has been used in other fields, use in dental offices has been limited. Chlorine dioxide may prove to be useful in dental disciplines. However, primarily because of the rapid deleterious effect on many metals, more clinical experience is necessary before results can be substantiated in the dental environment.

Summary

Choosing and using efficacious chemical sterilants and disinfectants in dentistry need not be confusing if a few important points are understood and observed:

1. The chemicals most appropriate for use in dentistry are mostly single purpose. No single chemical should be expected to satisfy all disinfection needs.

2. Heat sterilization should be used whenever possible because it is faster and more "error-proof" than liquid sterilization. Liquid sterilants are a compromise and should be used for sterilization only when a heat or heat/pressure system is not practical, such as with temperature sensitive plastic items.

3. Only liquid chemicals appropriately registered with the EPA or FDA should be used for disinfection/sterilization. ADA acceptance of a product identifies a properly registered product as appropriate for the dental environment.

4. All chemicals must be used in strict accordance with the registered instructions on the label. Any claims differing from, or in addition to, those on the label should be questioned.

5. The only "cold sterilizing" solutions readily available in dentistry are 2% glutaraldehydes, which must be used undiluted for the manufacturer's prescribed 6¾ to 10 hours, and chlorine dioxides. All other chemical products available in dentistry are disinfectants.

6. Glutaraldehydes are the most proven efficacious liquid chemicals for room-temperature sterilization; chlorine dioxides may prove to be useful specialty disinfectants and sterilants; iodophors are the most efficacious and practical surface disinfectants; and dilute glutaraldehydes and a new phenolic compound are the most efficacious room-temperature liquid instrument disinfectants. The new phenolic compound is the most efficacious holding (pre-cleaning) solution.

7. Quaternary ammonium compounds and alcohols are not effective and are not properly registered for dental disinfection and should not be used.

8. An antimicrobial soap containing appropriate concentrations of iodophor, PCMX, or chlorhexidine gluconate should be used for hand washing. Periodic application of one of the latter two chemical soaps between washings will maintain residual microbial reduction on the hands. An antimicrobial cream/lotion should be used with antimicrobial soaps to complete handcare.

As dental disciplines are increasingly identified and publicized as possible offenders in the transmission of new, emerging infectious diseases, knowledge of and correct utilization of chemical sterilants and disinfectants in dentistry will become increasingly important to the health of dental patients and dental personnel.

An efficacious program of cleaning-disinfecting includes careful cleaning of all items and surfaces to be treated; selection of properly registered and efficacious solution; and application of fresh solution to the cleaned surfaces. Manufacturers' recommendations should be carefully observed.

Disinfecting Surfaces

Historically, dental schools have taught students to disinfect surfaces and equipment by wetting a two-by-two gauze sponge with ethyl or isopropyl alcohol and then wiping certain items with the sponge. Often only one or two sponges are used, and after a few wipes, the small two-by-two sponges may be saturated with contaminated saliva and blood. Many studies have shown this technique to be inadequate and have shown, in fact, that the process may actually contribute to contamination by spreading the saliva and blood to surfaces which may have been previously untouched.

Much more effective disinfection is accomplished by using four-by-four gauze sponges, open cell plastic foam sponges or disposable toweling material which have been thoroughly wet with an effective disinfectant. Sponges used on grossly contaminated items should be discarded after very limited use. It is much better to use too many sponges than too few.

The first step in disinfection is cleaning grossly contaminated material from the surfaces. Sponges or toweling saturated with dilute iodophor or hypochlorite may be used for the "first" cleaning. A second application of the liquid agent is necessary for the actual disinfecting. The first application of the disinfecting solution may be "neutralized" by the presence of organic debris.

Disinfection of large, flat surfaces, such as counter tops and bracket tables, may be accomplished easily by spraying the surface with the disinfectant compound from a spray bottle. (See caution on the following page.) Sprayed surfaces should then be wiped with gauze, foam sponges or disposable toweling which have been wet with the disinfectant, to make certain the full surface has been covered. Excess disinfectant should be left in crevices, hard-to-clean corners, recesses, and depressions to ensure complete coverage of the possible contamination.

Surface disinfectants should be used only when the use of disposable barriers is impractical. THE MOST EFFECTIVE MICROBIAL BARRIER IS A DISPOSABLE COVER.

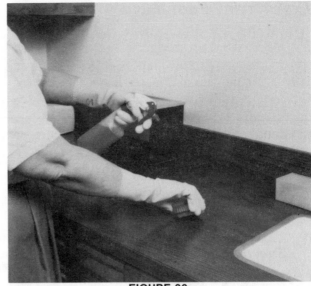

FIGURE 30
Spray to clean.

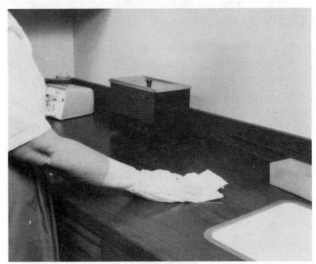

FIGURE 31
Clean and wipe.

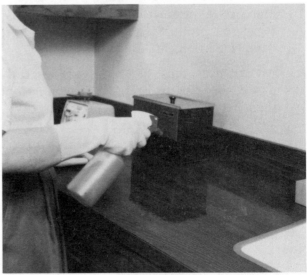

FIGURE 32

98   Spray to disinfect. Handles, switches, etc., should be wiped rather than sprayed.

Disinfecting Equipment

Handpieces, prophy angles, syringes, ultrasonic scaler tips, and other small, removable items (in addition to instruments) exposed to direct patient contact should be sterilized routinely. Sterilization of large immovable equipment in dental offices is not possible at present. Proper handling of this equipment, following patient treatment, requires use of an effective disinfectant. The same procedures and chemicals used on flat surfaces can be applied to disinfection of equipment. Disinfection is quickly accomplished by using a disinfectant spray followed by the saturated four-by-four gauze, plastic foam sponge, or disposable toweling technique previously described.

It should be noted that, while the use of the spray-wipe technique has become routine in many offices, several researchers have expressed reservations about the use of the spray mode. The possibility that aerosols may be created in the office raises the concern that respiratory complications may develop in personnel breathing the confined aerosols over a long period of time. Until further studies are done, personnel should be aware of this concern.

An interesting variation of the standard disinfection wipe technique was developed by Clinical Research Associates.[30] They used glutaraldehyde and suggested the following protocol:

> We suggest that the glutaraldehyde wrap technique might be used on equipment that is difficult to decontaminate, such as items that are too large to be immersed in disinfectant containers and such as pieces of equipment that are attached to stationary equipment. For clinical use, the technique we suggest is to wrap the object in a moistened gauze sponge of a convenient size, insert the gauze-wrapped object into a plastic bag, and secure the open end to retain moisture on the gauze for the desired amount of time. Use of protective covering for the hands is necessary because alkaline glutaraldehyde causes a temporary discoloration of human skin.

Equipment and items to be disinfected after each use include:

- Chair arms and headrest**
- Chair switches***
- Cuspidor bowl
- Handpieces*
- Handpiece holders
- Handpiece tubings
- HVE tip holder
- HVE tubings
- Light handles**
- Medicament bottles
- Nitrous masks*
- Nitrous tubings and surfaces*
- Operating stool arms and activator
- Saliva ejector holder and tubing
- Sink faucets, handles or levers
- Syringe*
- Syringe tubing*
- Unit arm
- Unit handles and switches
- X-ray head**
- X-ray switch**
- Pens, pencils, etc.

   * = if not sterilizable
   ** = unless covered with disposable barrier
   *** = unless foot controls are used.

In addition to the items listed above, any other item or part of equipment touched or contaminated with saliva, blood, or splatter must also be disinfected. WHEN IN DOUBT, CLEAN AND DISINFECT. It is very important to conscientiously clean and cover all surfaces with disinfectant, most particularly crevices, joints, depressions, and add-ons, where microbes are shielded.

Disposables

Many routinely used items, such as saliva ejectors, HVE tips and syringe needles, are available as inexpensive, single-use disposables. Use of disposables is preferred because the possibility of cross-contamination is lessened and clean-up is fast and easy. Cost of the items discarded is compensated by the saving of time for auxiliaries.

Even though some disposable items appear to have the possibility of re-use, studies have shown a high rate of infection from re-using disposables.[31] For this reason, the Food and Drug Administration has strong regulations regarding re-use of such items. Risks of re-use far outweigh minor savings from recirculation of disposables.

Many disposables are not packaged as pre-sterilized units but are supplied in industrially clean bulk with a number of units in each container. Industrially clean items are acceptable for use when pre-sterilized units are not indicated. While there may always be some risk of infection when sterile items are not used, studies have shown that industrial clean-packaging minimizes the possibility of infection.

Care must be exercised not to contaminate the remaining disposables when one is removed from the container. Use of sterile transfer forceps for removing the item to be used will minimize the possibility of contamination.

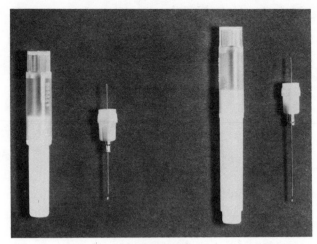

FIGURE 34
Disposable needles.

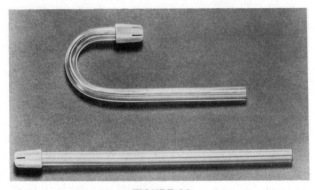

FIGURE 33
Disposable saliva ejectors.

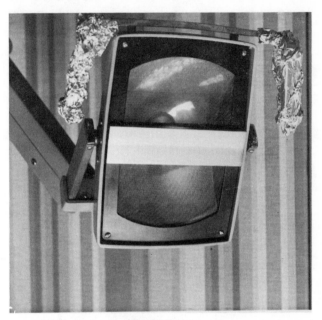

FIGURE 35
Disposable foil barrier on light handles.

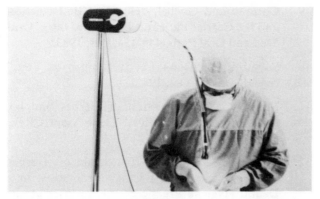

FIGURE 36
Disposable polyethylene barrier on fiber optic light.

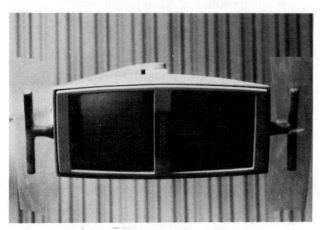

FIGURE 37
Disposable tubing on light handles.

Disposable covers, or barriers, should be used on light handles, chair arms and headrest, bracket table, x-ray head and yolk, and any other equipment which cannot be effectively disinfected. Some commercial, pre-formed covers are available. Bulk paper, aluminum foil or plastic sheet may also be used. While the bulk type covers may look a little cluttered to patients, prevention of cross-contamination is far more important. Explaining the reason for using bulk type covers may, in fact, impress certain patients with the care being taken to protect them from infection.

Waste Disposal

Surface-flush, "hidden" waste disposal container are much better than floor-open type or alligator type waste receptacles. Closed receptacles prevent air movement and prevent spreading contaminants. The receptacle should be lined with a plastic bag which can be removed without the removers touching the interior of either the container or the liner. The plastic bags should be changed frequently depending on the number and type of patients being treated. The bags should always be changed after treating a high risk patient, after each surgical procedure, or after each long operative procedure where a large amount of waste is generated. Without exception, waste bags should be changed daily, even in areas of very low usage, such as the x-ray or examining rooms. Moist waste material offers an ideal environment for the growth of microbes.

The instrument recirculation center should have a large capacity receptacle, since much of the waste from the treatment areas will be disposed of in the center.

All waste bags must be sealed before disposal and should be incinerated whenever possible. The possibility of infecting the general public through thoughtless waste disposal is very real. Many commercial waste collection services will not pick up at hospitals and clinics unless the waste is safely containerized.

Used needles should be bent or destroyed before disposal. Destruction without touching the needle is preferred. If needles are bent before disposal, care should be exercised by the person handling the needle not to nick or cut fingers. Small units are commercially available which mechanicaly destroy needles. (See Figure 38.) The used needles may also be placed in a container, covered with excess model plaster, and thereby rendered unusable. It is not unusual for drug users to search through hospital, clinic, and office waste for needles which are still usable. Needles and surgical blades should not be disposed of in plastic waste bags, since sharp edges may puncture the bags and allow leakage of contaminated waste.

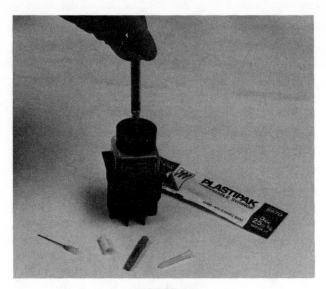

FIGURE 38
Needle disposing unit.

References and Suggested Readings

1. Bond, W.W., *et al.* "Inactivation of Hepatitis B Virus by Intermediate-to-High Level Disinfectant Chemicals." J Clin Micro 18:535-538, 1983.

2. Matis, *et al.* "Studies of Various Ultrasonic Cleaners." USAF School of Aerospace Medicine, Texas, 1980.

3. Schaefer, M. PRACTICAL INFECTION CONTROL IN THE DENTAL OFFICE, Sept, 1985.

4. Lyon, T.C. "Quaternary Ammonia Compounds: Should They Be Used for Disinfection in the Dental Office?" Oral Surg, 769-775, Nov, 1973.

5. American Dental Association. "Clinical Products in Dentistry—A Desk Top Reference." Jnl Am Dent Assn, Nov, 1984.

6. Dental Products Report. "Infection Control Report." Dec, 1985.

7. Clinical Research Associates. "Use Survey—1985." 9:8, Aug, 1985.

8. American Dental Association, Council on Dental Therapeutics. "Quaternary Ammonium Compounds Not Acceptable for Disinfection of Instruments on Environmental Surfaces in Dentistry." Jnl of Am Dent Assn, 97:844-856, Nov, 1978.

9. Cottone and Goebel. "Hepatitis B: Detection and the Carrier Patient." Jnl of Oral Surg, Oral Med and Oral Path, 449-454, Oct, 1983.

10. Sabatini, B. "Don't Let It Happen to You." NADL Jnl, 19, Oct, 1982.

11. Miller, C. "Transmission of Herpes Simplex Virus in a Dental Office." Dent Asepsis Rev, 5:11, Nov, 1984.

12. Manzella, *et al.* "An Outbreak of Herpes Simplex Virus Type 1 Gingivostomatitis, in a Dental Hygiene Practice." Jnl Am Med Assn, 252:15, 19-22, Oct, 1984.

13. Conte, J.E., Jr.; Hadley, W.K.; and Sande, M. Task force. "Infection Control Guidelines for Patients with the Acquired Immunodeficiency Syndrome (AIDS)." New Engl Jnl Med 309: 740-744, 1983.

14. Neumann, H.H. "When is AIDS Communicable?" JAMA 251:1553, 1984.

15. Crawford, J.J. "Sterilization, Disinfection and Asepsis in Dentistry." *In* Block, S.S., ed. DISINFECTION, STERILIZATION AND PRESERVATION, ed 3. Philadelphia, Lea & Febiger, 505-523, 1983.

16. Crawford, J.J. "State-of-the-Art: Practical Infection Control in Dentistry." Hepatitis Symposium, 10:629-633, JADA, Apr, 1983.

17. *Op cit,* ADA.

18. *Op cit,* ADA.

19. Johnson & Johnson. CIDEX glutaraldehyde product label, 1985.

20. Environmental Protection Agency, Registration Division, 1987.

21. Favero, M.S. "Iodine-Champagne in a Tin Cup." Infec Cont, 3:1, 30-32, 1982.

22. *Op cit*, Bond.

23. *Op cit*, Favero.

24. *Op cit*, Crawford.

25. Dexide, Inc. "Summary of Safety and Effectiveness Data—ULTRADEX Surgical Hand Scrub." 1984.

26. American Dental Association, Council on Dental Therapeutics, Acceptance Guidelines, 1980.

27. American Dental Association, Council on Dental Therapeutics. "Acceptance of Disinfectant for Instruments and Equipment." Jnl Am Dent Assn, 110:394, Mar, 1985.

28. *Ibid.*

29. *Ibid.*

30. Christensen, R. "Effectiveness of Glutaraldehyde as a Chemosterilizer Used in a Wrapping Technique on Simulated Metal Instruments," July, 1977. Clin Res Assoc, Jnl of Dent Res, 822-826.

31. FDA, One-Use Disposable Guidelines, 1981.

Chapter Seven
REVIEW EXERCISES

Date _____Name_____

Circle the letters of the terms which most closely approximate the answers. There may be one or more than one correct answer. If you circle D, indicate the other answer or answers, if known.

1. The most important step in disinfection is:

   A. choosing the right disinfectant

   B. pre-cleaning

   C. using enough disinfectant

   D. other_____

2. Effectiveness of a disinfectant is determined partly by:

   A. biocidal activity

   B. user technique

   C. room temperature

   D. other_____

3. The American Dental Association will not accept a disinfectant of:

   A. iodophor

   B. quaternary ammonium

   C. alcohol

   D. other_____

4. Disinfectants are used for two primary reasons in dentistry:

   A. to disinfect and sterilize

   B. to disinfect heat sensitive items and surfaces

   C. to disinfect equipment and cabinets

   D. other_____

5. The American Dental Association and the Centers for Disease Control have suggested the use of several disinfectants, including:

   A. alcohol and glutaraldehyde

   B. iodophor and alcohol

   C. dilute iodophor and sodium hypochlorite

   D. other_____

6. The most practical dental surface disinfectant is a dilution of:

A. alcohol and glutaraldehyde

B. iodophor and alcohol

C. iodophor or phenolic compounds

D. other_____

7. The most common historical surface disinfection technique includes the use of:

A. heavy rubber gloves

B. paper towel and alcohol-iodophor

C. 2 x 2 gauze and alcohol

D. other_____

8. A preferable surface disinfection technique includes the use of:

A. cloth towel and alcohol-iodophor

B. phenol spray

C. 4 x 4 gauze or foam sponge iodophor or phenolic

D. other_____

9. Large surfaces may be disinfected by the use of:

A. spray-wipe-spray technique

B. disinfectant flood technique

C. wipe and dry technique

D. other_____

10. All small equipment, such as handpieces, should be:

A. sterilized whenever possible

B. disassembled before sterilization

C. disassembled before disinfection

D. other_____

11. Items to be disinfected after each patient include:

A. cuspidor bowl

B. sink

C. light

D. other_____

12. The use of disposables rather than metal items on patients is good because:

A. they are inexpensive

B. there is less chance of contamination

C. they are not cold to the patient's mouth

D. other_____

13. Disposables are sometimes packaged:

A. in bulk   B. industrially clean   C. pre-sterilized

D. other_____

14. Disposable barriers should be used on:

A. light handles   B. cuspidor bowls   C. HVE hoses

D. other_____

15. Surface disinfectants should be used:

A. to sterilize cabinets   B. when the use of disposable barriers is impractical   C. in place of heat sterilizers

D. other_____

16. The preferred waste disposal container is:

A. floor-open   B. alligator type   C. hidden surface-flush

D. other_____

17. Plastic disposable waste liners should be changed:

A. at least daily   B. weekly   C. after every high risk patient

D. other_____

18. Used needles should be disposed of by:

A. sealing in plastic bags   B. sealing in plaster   C. inserting in cotton roll

D. other_____

NOTE: Answers to the review exercises appear in the back of this book.

Is It Legal?

ABSTRACT: Chemical disinfectants and sterilants are subject to certain Federal laws and other regulations and guidelines. It is very important that manufacturers, distributors, recommenders, AND ALL DENTAL PERSONNEL have a knowledge of such laws, regulations, and guidelines.

Proper observance of the legalities of disinfectants and sterilants assures efficacious usage and minimized exposure to malpractice actions.

Readers may question the need for a discussion of legalities and regulatory compliance in a book on infectious disease. With the present dynamics of dental infection control, catalyzed by the "Hudson Syndrome," the announcement that Mr. Rock Hudson had AIDS, it is very important to recognize that the practice of efficacious infection control and a working knowledge of regulatory and advisory laws and guidelines are inseparable.

The potential transmission of infectious diseases and the practice of procedures for the control of such diseases is becoming more challenging to dentistry at the same time that the public is becoming increasingly aware of dentistry's role in infectious disease transmission.

Also, manufacturers are developing new generations of infection control products and systems which are being introduced in increasing numbers through several channels of distribution. Because of the highly technical aspects of some of the products and systems, some of the information has become confusing to many persons in dentistry.

Some of the reasons for the confusion are as follows:

1. Some professional and auxiliary schools in dentistry do not provide the latest information on infection control procedures or the latest information on the most efficacious products and systems for control of infectious diseases.

2. Industry is rapidly developing new, more effective products, and the complexities of such products occasionally result in distortions of product information as the products move from marketing to distribution to the end user. Often conflicting or misunderstood claims make it difficult for most dental personnel to separate fact from fiction.

3. Several agencies are responsible for registration, enforcement, and acceptance under laws/guidelines for infection control. For instance, the Environmental Protection Agency (EPA) is primarily responsible for administering Federal law regulating disinfectants and sterilants for use on inanimate surfaces and objects. The Food and Drug Administration (FDA) is responsible for administering Federal law regulating skin antimicrobials, including hand scrubs, skin preps,

hand washes, and antiseptics. And the American Dental Association (ADA) develops and administers guidelines for an acceptance program for both categories of products.

To add further complexity, Underwriter's Laboratories, Inc. (UL) and the American Society of Mechanical Engineers (ASME) are also involved in certain aspects of the regulatory compliance for equipment and machines.

4. In some instances, regulatory and advisory agencies have not updated specifications and guidelines at the same rate that products have evolved. As an illustration, neither the EPA nor the ADA presently separates immersion and environmental surface disinfectants into different categories in their registration/acceptance programs, as many experts feel is necessary. The ADA is presently considering separation of these categories.[1]

5. Dental professionals and staff often resist change from traditional techniques and products. For example, A MAJORITY OF DENTAL PERSONNEL STILL USE QUATERNARY AMMONIUM COMPOUNDS AND ALCOHOLS FOR DISINFECTION, EVEN THOUGH SUCH PRODUCTS HAVE BEEN NOT RECOMMENDED FOR USE IN DENTISTRY BY ALL REGULATORY AGENCIES AND MOST RESEARCHERS FOR MANY YEARS.[2][3]

6. Some infectious disease experts, with understandably limited experience and knowledge in the regulatory field, present programs, including recommendations of products, without referencing the need to consider regulatory compliance. Improper use of the products can result in malpractice suits if patient infection results. As an example, the use of combinations of chemicals has been recommended for disinfection of environmental surfaces even though the chemicals are not registered with the EPA as inanimate disinfectants, as required under the FIFR Act.[4]

Further, research groups occasionally publish data comparing the effectiveness of skin products to the effectiveness of properly registered products for disinfection of environmental surfaces. The data is published without explaining or referencing the regulatory and legal implications of the improper use of such products, or the use of legally acceptable products used in an illegal manner.

The two examples cited are presently occurring, and the result of the actions of the experts and the researchers may be to inadvertently encourage the use of potentially illegal products. *THE ISSUE IS NOT ONLY ONE OF EFFICACY BUT ALSO ONE OF LAW AND THE POTENTIAL INVOLVEMENT OF ALL PARTIES IN OFTEN DEVASTATING MALPRACTICE SUITS.* Persons advocating use of products must be cautious in their recommendations. With the increased public awareness of potential transmission of infectious diseases in dental environments, more malpractice suits will be filed involving dental personnel *AND* companies or persons who knowingly or unwittingly violate existing laws, or encourage violation by others, of existing laws.

DENTISTS, HYGIENISTS, STAFF, AND OTHER PERSONS IN DENTISTRY MUST HAVE A WORKING KNOWLEDGE OF INFECTION CONTROL REGULATORY REQUIREMENTS TO ASSURE USE OF ONLY THE MOST EFFICACIOUS PRODUCTS AND TO MINIMIZE THE POSSIBILITY OF ACCIDENTAL INVOLVEMENT IN MALPRACTICE SUITS.

The EPA and the FIFR Act

The Federal Insecticide, Fungicide, and Rodenticide Act (FIFR Act) became U.S. Federal law in 1947 and dealt mainly with the use of insecticides and pesticides, some of which, until the adoption of this Act, had been misused by industry and the farming community. The Act was amended in 1962 to expand regulation to a number of "non-insecticide" chemicals, including certain healthcare disinfectants and sterilants. Under the FIFR Act, the EPA registers all *CHEMICALS* intended to be used as disinfectants and sterilants on inanimate objects or surfaces.

The registration procedures are exacting and demanding, requiring—in the case of sterilants—the 100% kill of 360 replicates containing hundreds of millions of resistant spores. The tests must then be repeated a second time with a 100% kill. If one replicate of the 720 tested survives, the product does not meet the criteria of a sterilant. Disinfectant tests, while still very stringent, do not require kill of resistant spores.

All disinfectants and sterilants must meet minimal standards. However, if manufacturers wish to claim kill of additional microbes, such as *Mycobacterium tuberculosis*, corroborating studies must be submitted for approval by EPA of the additional claims.

Also, the EPA reviews toxicological and hazards data, product literature, and other company data. A successful registration takes many months, costs thousands of dollars, and results in issuance of a *REGISTRATION NUMBER TO BE DISPLAYED ON THE LABEL AS EVIDENCE THAT THE PRODUCT IS LEGALLY REGISTERED FOR SALE IN INTERSTATE COMMERCE AS A DISINFECTANT OR STERILANT.* The number appears on the label as EPA Registration No. XXXXXXXX, which is evidence of compliance with requirements of the FIFR Act.

The FIFR Act serves a useful purpose. However, the Act may also contribute to confusion because the EPA regulates only with *CHEMICAL* sterilants and disinfectants. Steam autoclaves and dry heat sterilizers are not regulated under the Act, and manufacturers of these two modes of sterilization are not subject to the same Federal scrutiny as are chemical systems manufacturers.

A section of the FIFR Act provides that anyone manufacturing, distributing, using, or recommending the use of *ANY CHEMICAL DISINFECTANT OR STERILANT* must comply with the terms of the Act or such persons are potentially in violation of Federal law.

The FIFR Act is very significant to all of dentistry. BECAUSE OF THE ACT, MANUFACTURERS CANNOT MAKE LEGAL CLAIMS FOR PRODUCTS BEYOND THOSE APPROVED BY THE EPA AND THE FDA. BECAUSE OF THE ACT, CLINICIANS AND RESEARCHERS CANNOT LEGALLY RECOMMEND THE USE OF PRODUCTS WHICH ARE NOT PROPERLY REGISTERED WITH EPA OR FDA. BECAUSE OF THE ACT, USERS MUST USE PRODUCTS IN ACCORDANCE WITH INSTRUCTIONS ON THE LABEL.

Finally and urgently, dental personnel must be aware of the FIFR Act because dental personnel who use an EPA registered product *OTHER THAN AS DIRECTED ON THE LABEL MAY HAVE COMMITTED A POTENTIALLY ILLEGAL ACT AND ARE SUBJECT TO THE LEGAL IMPLICATIONS THEREOF IF SOMEONE IS INJURED BY THE IMPROPER USE, AS IN THE CASE OF A PATIENT WHO ACQUIRES AN INFECTIOUS DISEASE.*

While the law has not been tested extensively in dentistry, indications suggest that the end user dentist, hygienist, or other staff will become increasingly responsible for misuse of products, when the misuse results in transmission of an infectious disease to patients.

It is very important that dental personnel understand the significance of the FIFR Act for at least two important reasons:

1. Choices of efficacious disinfectants and sterilants become easier and less confusing if the significance of statements on the label of the products are fully understood. Asking product representatives for answers to regulatory questions is a valuable aid in assessing the knowledge of the representative and in eliciting conscientious responses.

2. Knowledge of some aspects of the law and compliance therewith may prove to be mandatory in successfully countering malpractice actions as a result of patient-acquired infectious diseases.

It is also important that persons teaching infection control understand the significance of the FIFR Act. Recommending the use by dental personnel of products which are not properly registered under the Act potentially places the recommender at risk of involvement in litigation if the recommendation leads to patient infection traceable to misuse of a product.

The FDA

Federal law provides for the Food and Drug Administration to register all products used on or in the human body. Depending on the type of product, notification without extensive testing may be all that is necessary. However, as in the case of disinfectants or sterilants, an evaluation process similar to that used by of the EPA is required by the FDA.

An NDC (National Drug Commission) number is issued upon satisfactory completion of the FDA registration process. Similar disclosure criteria apply, and only claims approved by the FDA may be used in sale of the product.

IN SUMMARY, AN EPA NUMBER ON A LABEL INDICATES THE PRODUCT MAY BE LEGALLY USED ONLY ON INANIMATE OBJECTS OR SURFACES, AND AN NDC NUMBER ON A LABEL INDICATES THE PRODUCT MAY BE LEGALLY USED ONLY ON OR IN THE BODY.

Table 11 on the following page suggests simple guidelines for determining efficiency and legality of chemical disinfectants and sterilants.

The ADA Acceptance Program

The ADA Product Acceptance Program provides guidelines for acceptance of certain infection control products. The ADA Program does not have the same legal implications as those under the FIFR Act or FDA registration. However, knowledge by dental personnel of the program is very important for judging product efficacy *for use in the dental environment*.

The ADA Council on Dental Therapeutics is responsible for evaluating all therapeutic agents used in the diagnosis, treatment, or *prevention of dental disease*. The acceptance program "evaluates the safety and efficacy of these agents, using laboratory and clinical data submitted by the manufacturer."[5] The program studies product submissions to determine *usefulness and safety of the product in the practice of dentistry*. Certain infection control products may have application in disciplines other than dentistry where microbiological challenges are less stringent. However, use of such "weaker" products is contraindicated in dentistry. ADA acceptance signifies that the product is acceptable for use in the dental environment.

Acceptance of a product under ADA guidelines includes the following criteria:

1. The product must be properly registered with all applicable U.S. governmental agencies, including the EPA and the FDA.

2. The product must be reviewed by one or more ADA consultants specializing in the product discipline. In the case of disinfectants and sterilants, one or more consultants are microbiologists.

3. The product must be reviewed for potential usefulness in dentistry. Independent studies supporting claims made for the product are often required before the application is submitted to the Council for final approval.

4. Acceptance of the product is granted only by vote of the members of The Council on Dental Therapeutics. Acceptance of the product may be evidenced by appropriately displaying the ADA Seal of Acceptance on the product and/or advertising materials.

TABLE 11

Suggested Guidelines for Choosing Efficacious and Legal Chemical Disinfectants, Sterilants and Antimicrobials

FOR USE ON INANIMATE SURFACES
(Instruments, Bracket Tables, Cabinets, Handpieces and Syringes, Tubings, Etc.)

1. Product label must display an EPA registration number.
2. Product must be used exactly as instructed ON THE EPA LABEL.
3. Product must claim to kill *Mycobacterium tuberculosis*.
4. Product should display the ADA Seal of Acceptance (optional).

FOR USE ON ANIMATE SURFACES
(Skin)

1. Product must display an NDC registration number.
2. Product must be used exactly as instructed ON THE FDA LABEL.
3. Product should claim to kill *Mycobacterium tuberculosis* (optional).

Summary

IN SUMMARY, KNOWLEDGE OF FEDERAL, STATE, AND PROFESSIONAL ORGANIZATION LAWS, REGULATIONS, AND/OR ADVISORY PROGRAMS EFFECTING DENTISTRY WILL BECOME MORE IMPORTANT TO ALL DENTAL PERSONNEL AS THE PROFESSION AND RELATED DISCIPLINES BECOME MORE VISIBLE IN THE FIELD OF INFECTIOUS DISEASES. REGULATORY COMPLIANCE RELATES TO POSSIBLE MALPRACTICE LEGAL ACTIONS. ADDITIONALLY, KNOWLEDGE OF SUCH PROGRAMS CONTRIBUTES TO CHOICES OF EFFICACIOUS PRODUCTS AND THEREBY TO EFFICACIOUS INFECTION CONTROL.

References and Suggested Readings

1. Burrell, K. American Dental Association, "Suggested New Guidelines." Coun on Dent Ther Adv Panel, Jan, 1986.

2. Lyon, T.C. "Quaternary Ammonia Compounds: Should They Be Used for Disinfection in the Dental Office?" Oral Surg, 769-775, Nov, 1973.

3. American Dental Association, Council on Dental Therapeutics. "Quaternary Ammonium Compounds Not Acceptable for Disinfection of Instruments on Environmental Surfaces in Dentistry." Jnl of Am Dent Assn, 97:844-856, Nov, 1978.

4. Federal Insecticide, Fungicide, and Rodenticide Act, 1947, amended 1962, amended 1978.

5. American Dental Association, Council on Dental Therapeutics. "Acceptance Guidelines." 1985.

Chapter Eight
REVIEW EXERCISES

Date _____ Name_____

Circle the letters of the terms which most closely approximate the answers. There may be one or more than one correct answer. If you circle D, indicate the other answer or answers, if known.

1. Federal agencies regulating liquid sterilants/disinfectants/skin antimicrobials include:

    A. EPA   B. FDA   C. FCC

    D. other_____

2. The FIFR Act is:

    A. a state law   B. a book on regulations C. a Federal law

    D. other_____

3. Under the FIFR Act, healthcare personnel must:

    A. use products wisely   B. use only registered products   C. advise patients of rights

    D. other_____

4. Skin antimicrobials are regulated by:

    A. ADA   B. EPA   C. FTC

    D. other_____

5. The ADA offers:

    A. free advice   B. samples of disinfectants   C. an Acceptance Program

    D. other_____

6. Healthcare professionals should choose certain regulated products by:

    A. observing certain guidelines   B. asking supplypersons   C. asking professors

    D. other_____

7. Use of non-efficacious products may result in:

   A. dismissal from office   B. suspension from work   C. malpractice action

   D. other_____

NOTE: Answers to the review exercises are in the back of this book.

Choosing and Using Sterilization Equipment and Supplies

ABSTRACT: Everything that can be sterilized must be sterilized and NOT in certain "cold sterilizing solutions" such as quaternary ammonium compounds.

There is no all-purpose sterilizer. The use of two or more of the generally accepted methods of dental sterilization may be indicated in a busy practice.

The use of certain aids with the sterilizer(s) completes the sterility assurance program.

An important part of patient treatment is the availability of sterilized instruments and items and the recirculation of these instruments and items after they have been used. The correct choice of the most practical sterilizer (or sterilizers) for use in dental instrument recirculation procedures is the heart of an infection control program. While it is always difficult, if not impossible, to name a "most important" item or action, sterilization of everything that can be sterilized may be the action "most important" to infection control.

Historically, dental sterilization methods have included boiling water and "cold sterilizing solutions." Neither method is acceptable, except for limited use of glutaraldehyde liquid sterilants. The "cold sterilizing solutions" normally referred to by personnel, and still in wide use in dentistry, are mostly quaternary ammonium compounds, even though the American Dental Association and many others have discouraged use of the chemical. Historical "COLD STERILIZING SOLUTIONS" ARE DISINFECTANTS AND ARE NOT STERILANTS and should not be used in place of true sterilants. Quaternary ammonium compounds are not recommended as sterilants nor disinfectants since their biocidal activity is far surpassed by certain other products (see Chapter 7). The biocidal activity of quaternary ammonium compounds is easily compromised by contamination with certain other materials, such as ordinary detergents.

Dentistry has been so deeply entrenched in the use of "cold sterilizing solutions" that it is difficult to convince some dentists of the necessity for using true sterilants for certain instruments and items. Even highly publicized studies, such as the work by the American Dental Association showing that quaternary ammonium compounds are not acceptable as disinfectants[1] seems to have had minimal impact on much of dentistry. Many offices continue to use cold disinfectants for items such as burs and cutting instruments, even when the same offices have heat/pressure sterilizers which could be used effectively and without harm to such instruments. LIQUID DISINFECTANTS ARE A COMPROMISE and must not be used, except for items which cannot be cycled in one or more of the generally accepted methods of sterilization.

As dental personnel and patients are becoming increasingly aware of infection control, more manufacturers and distributors are offering greater choices of sterilization equipment. As a consequence, choosing sterilization equipment has become somewhat confusing.

One reason for the confusion is that not all methods of sterilization fall under regulatory control. In the United States, the Environmental Protection Agency and the American Dental Association study, register, or accept all forms of chemical sterilization, including glutaraldehydes, chemical vapor sterilizers, and ethylene oxide sterilizers. The EPA regulations and testing are very specific and very difficult. Included in the EPA regulatory process is a review of all technical software and advertising literature to make certain that claims made for the products are accurate and supported by scientific data. An EPA registration number on a product is assurance that the product works as represented when used according to the manufacturer's instructions.

Autoclaves and dry heat sterilizers are not regulated by the EPA because they are not considered chemical sterilizers. The ADA Council on Dental Materials, Instruments and Equipment has an Acceptance Program for autoclave sterilizers. The ADA is working in conjunction with American National Standards Institute and the International Standards Organization to establish specifications and standards for all sterilizers. At the present time, it is necessary for purchasers to conduct their own investigation before making final decisions on which sterilizer or sterilizers to purchase.

Another source of confusion in choosing a sterilizer for purchase is the level of expertise of the manufacturer in producing, testing, and developing accurate claims for the equipment. Some products are nearly always efficacious, and are usually accompanied by complete and useful owner and operator instructions making statements supported by well-documented studies. Conversely, other companies with little or no special expertise, offer products which are not always fully proven or tested. For example, several types of ultra-violet sterilizers have been sold in dentistry. Ultra-violet rays will sterilize if the microorganisms are exposed and if they are in the direct line of the rays. However, ultra-violet rays cannot penetrate dense or opaque materials; therefore, ultra-violet sterilization is impractical for dental use.

Another example of unsupported claims has been evidenced over the past few years in several European countries where a "sterilizer" has become somewhat popular. This "sterilizer" is an ultrasonic cleaner with an ultra-violet lid which functions when the cleaner is turned on. The manufacturer claims that the ultrasonic action "floats" the microbes to the surface where the ultra-violet rays accomplish 100 percent kill. Such a claim is ridiculous to persons knowledgeable in sterilization, and yet hundreds of the units were sold until a respected German university recently studied the unit and disputed the manufacturer's claims. Even so, the unit is still being sold in limited numbers in the countries where there is no regulation of sterilization.

Finally, at this writing there are several products being sold to dental offices in the United States which are impractical or potentially dangerous. One product is manufactured by the Anprolene Company and is a small ethylene canister which vents residuals directly into the room when the canister is opened by the operator. Ethylene oxide has been shown to be a mutagen and a potential carcinogen, and use of the chemical in this manner is in direct violation of FDA guidelines for the handling of ethylene oxide sterilants. Certain other products, while not particularly dangerous, are not practical for general office use. For example, a system in which glutaraldehyde must be heated in an ultrasonic device requires special equipment for use, and the heating process increases the vapor toxicity activity.

How then should a sterilizer be chosen for the dental office? First, the dentist should familiarize himself or herself with proven methods of sterilization by reading publications from the American Dental Association, the U.S. Pharmacopoeia, the Public Health Service, the U.S. Medical Material Board, the U.S. Air Force School of Aerospace Medicine, the U.S. Navy, and other sources.

Once a reasonable representation of the scientific sterilizer information has been assimilated, the dentist should compile a list of the sterilization needs of the office. This list will serve to establish the final parameters for selecting the sterilizer or sterilizers. After establishing parameters, the dentist should ask persons in the dental field, including experienced practitioners and knowledgeable supply salesmen, for their recommendations of the best equipment available within his or her parameters. It is very important, however, to test these recommendations against published data, since practitioners and supply persons are not always experts in sterilization.

Finally, the dentist should make a considered, intelligent, and personal decision based on the information gathered in the studies. This procedure may seem arduous, time-consuming, and somewhat complicated, but the exercise is absolutely necessary because the sterilizer(s) is the heart of the infection control program.

Establishing Parameters

The process of selecting a sterilizer(s) should include answering at least the following questions:

1. How fast are instruments to be turned around each day?

2. How many patients will be seen each day?

3. Will the items to be sterilized be predominantly textiles, instruments, water, chemicals, or combinations thereof?

4. What kind of instruments will be used most frequently—burs, files, reamers, surgical forceps, periodontal instruments, orthodontic instruments?

5. How many disposables will be used?

6. What kind of packaging will be used?

The answers to these and other questions will serve to establish parameters to help determine the category or method of sterilization most appropriate for the office.

Four Categories of Sterilizers

There are four generally accepted categories of sterilizers (see Table 12). Ethylene oxide sterilant is not included in this comparison since studies have shown ethylene oxide to be potentially mutagenic and carcinogenic. Recent guidelines issued by the Food and Drug Administration place strict limitations on the use of ethylene oxide sterilant. These limitations make the use of ethylene oxide impractical in all but the most controlled environments, such as hospitals. Dental offices, clinics, and schools should not consider using ethylene oxide unless they are prepared for a demanding commitment to protection of staff and patients from the gas residuals.

The use of sterilizers which are not included in the four generally accepted categories should be questioned very seriously. While development of new technology is inevitable and desirable, advancements must be well-tested and well-documented before they are accepted for general use. Office experimentation should be conducted only under a well-designed and controlled program to assure protection of the health of patients and personnel.

Dry Heat Sterilization

Of the four generally accepted methods of dental sterilization, dry heat has the lowest initial cost. Routine operating cost is also low as long as care is taken to avoid damaging high-heat sensitive instruments and items. Maintenance is minimal because the units are of simple construction and contain a minimum of moving parts.

Dry heat sterilizers provide an acceptable method of sterilization for offices where instrument turn-around time is not a primary concern and where such offices have an alternative method of sterilization for high-heat sensitive instruments and items.

Dry heat may be the least practical of the heat methods for busy dental offices because of the relatively long instrument turn-around time. Dry heat sterilizers require two hours at 320 degrees

TABLE 12

FOUR GENERALLY ACCEPTED METHODS OF DENTAL STERILIZATION					
Method	Temperature	Time	Approximate Cost	Advantages—	Disadvantages
Autoclave	250°-275°F. 121°-134°C.	15-40 minutes plus drying time.	$1,200.00 to $3,000.00 plus deionized water.	Excellent penetration. Best for textiles, water, culture media, chemical solutions.	Rusts, dulls, corrodes certain metals, especially carbon steel. Loads wet on completion.
Chemical Vapor Sterilizer	270°F. 132°C.	20 minutes plus rise time	$1,400.00 to $2,900.00 plus solution	Water content below rust, dulling, corrosion threshold—will not harm metals. Loads come out dry.	Slow penetration—not good for heavier loads of textiles, chemicals, water or culture media. Special solution required. Good ventilation or filtration required.
Dry Heat	320°F. 160°C.	2 hours	$400.00 to $900.00	Inexpensive. Low maintenance. Best for glassware and dry chemicals.	Length of cycle long. Instruments must be separated carefully or will not sterilize. Melts or destroys certain metal and solder joints.
Glutaraldehyde	Ambient	6¾ hours to 10 hours	$500.00 to $600.00 per year average use	Sterilizes "low temperature" items which would be destroyed in heat systems. Low initial cost.	Shortens sterility time. Certain kinds discolor hands. Sterile packaging not possible. Rinse with sterile water after use. Limited life. Expensive on continuous use basis. Will rust instruments if left in too long. No way to monitor sterility.
Glutaraldehyde Oxide	60°C 140°F.	1 Hr.	plus cost of a "dedicated" heating unit.		

fahrenheit for a complete cycle. Since temperatures above 300 degrees fahrenheit begin to damage certain metals and materials, items are limited which can be placed in dry heat without damage. For example, solder joints on impression trays and certain other items begin to break down at approximately 300 degrees fahrenheit, and cutting edges on certain "sharp" instruments are destroyed with repetitive cycling above 335 degrees fahrenheit. It is important to operate dry heat sterilizers at the lowest possible temperature and for the longest period of time which still assure dependable sterilization.

If one is in doubt concerning potential damage to instruments, one should consult manufacturers of the instruments for information concerning the effects of dry heat sterilization. Hu-Friedy, a manufacturer of dental instruments, has acknowledged problems with instruments cycled in excessively high heat sterilizers.

They print the following disclaimer on all instrument packaging:

> NOTICE: INSPECT AND STERILIZE THIS INSTRUMENT PRIOR TO EACH USE. This package contains a delicate, hand-crafted dental instrument. Use it only for its intended purpose to insure its effectiveness and maximum life. Proper care must be given during cleaning, sharpening and sterilization procedures to preserve design and integrity and to prolong its usefulness. All conventional methods of cleaning and sterilization are acceptable. However, higher than recommended chemical concentrations and/or sterilization temperatures (270-345 F.) in excess of normal may result in premature instrument failure.

Dry heat standards in Germany and Switzerland require use of a temperature of 180 C. because of inconsistent sterilization below that level.

In addition to time and temperature limitations, dry heat tends to stratify air, thereby creating pockets where sterilization may not be accomplished. Also, most table-top dry heat sterilizers utilize convection heating; therefore, heat distri-

bution may be irregular, resulting in a substantial variation in temperatures within the sterilization chamber. Stratification and temperature variation can be partially controlled by using fan-forced air circulation in the unit and by careful insulation of the chamber and the door of the unit. Dry heat sterilizers must be loaded carefully and loosely to assure maximum hot air penetration around instruments. (See Figure 39.)

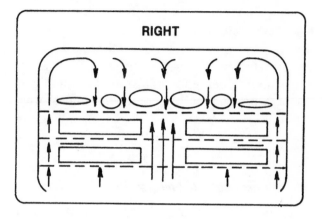

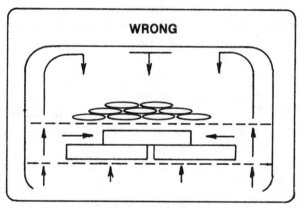

FIGURE 39
Illustration of correct way to load dry heat sterilizers to assure proper heat circulation.

The use of non-dental, commercial baking ovens has occasionally been suggested for dental sterilization. In such cases, it is pointed out that the ovens must be equipped with thermisters to check the adequacy of temperatures. While this approach to sterilization may be acceptable in practices where the dentist is deeply involved in the procedures and the monitoring of sterility, such an approach is not acceptable for most offices. As previously stated, dental dry heat sterilizers must be used carefully to assure sterility. Introducing additional variables by hand-making sterilizers from equipment not designed for sterilization is potentially dangerous and may be difficult to defend in case of a malpractice suit. It is much better to purchase sterilizers designed, constructed, and warranted by reputable manufacturers and capable of being serviced by knowledgeable dental dealer personnel.

Instruments must be dry when placed in dry heat; otherwise rust and corrosion may result. Instruments and items should be packaged in trays or foil wrappings. Paper and cloth wraps will usually char and/or disintegrate at higher temperatures, thereby compromising storage capability.

Glutaraldehyde Sterilization

Two percent glutaraldehyde chemicals have come into limited use in only the past decade. One of the reasons given by practitioners for using glutaraldehydes for sterilization in place of one of the heat sterilants is low cost. A 1982 study done at Baylor University[2] has shown that the cost of using glutaraldehyde sterilants is nearly six hundred dollars per year. This figure does not take into account additional equipment or supplies, such as trays and sterile water. The cost of glutaraldehydes varies with each product, but none can be considered inexpensive.

Glutaraldehydes are liquid chemicals available in several forms, including alkaline, acidic, phenolic-buffered, and heat-potentiated. Depending on the form, sterility is achieved in 6¾ to 10 hours, and disinfection is achieved in approximately ten minutes. The heat potentiated form requires a temperature of approximately 60 degrees centigrade and has several disadvantages, including odor, increased toxicity, and incompatability with certain metals.[3] All glutaraldehydes do not have the same physical characteristics, and some are more practical for use in dental offices than others. As with other methods of sterilization, it is important to secure and read independent scientific data when selecting a glutaraldehyde.

Glutaraldehydes should be used primarily for sterilizing temperature-sensitive materials, such as low temperature plastic and fiber optic devices, and they may be used as "holding solutions" until contaminated instruments can be cleaned. Practical use of glutaraldehydes as a sterilant is limited because of (1) the extended time required for sterilization, (2) the necessity to raise the temperature for efficacy of acidic glutaraldehydes, (3) the fact that instruments cannot be prepackaged for storage, and, most important, (4) the fact that there is no way to monitor sterility-efficacy on a routine basis. Some manufacturers offer color indicator devices which change when less than one percent glutaraldehyde remains.

Claims made by certain manufacturers for glutaraldehydes can be confusing. Some literature, for example, states that certain vegetative microorganisms are sterilized in ten minutes while spores take hours to kill. The directions for use do not describe how to separate the vegetative microbes from the spores to allow utilization of the shorter time. Unfortunately, there is no practical way to know which organisms are present. Therefore, since STERILE is a very specific term meaning that all microorganisms are destroyed each and every time, the longer time must always be used to achieve sterility.

Steam Autoclave Sterilization

The steam autoclave is the oldest and best known of the generally accepted dental sterilization methods, having been invented by Chamberland,[4] a pupil of Pasteur, in 1873. Commonly accepted parameters for autoclaving are 121 degrees centigrade and fifteen pounds per square inch pressure for fifteen to 40 minutes of exposure to the saturated steam. The longer times are usually necessary to assure penetration of heavy loads of textiles. Shorter periods of time at higher temperatures, sometimes called "flash" sterilization, are also possible. "Flash" sterilization is a term used to describe cycling at a temperature of 132-135 degrees centigrade for three to five minutes. "Flash" sterilization should be used mainly for sterilizing a few instruments or items which are needed in an "emergency" turn-around. The shortened sterilization time of "flashing" involves more operator judgment and leaves little margin for error.

Pressurized steam in a pre-evacuated chamber offers the advantage of quick penetration by the sterilant through the packaging to the items to be sterilized. Also, spores are killed more quickly in the presence of moisture. Moist heat/pressure systems kill through a process of denaturation, while dry heat systems kill through the longer process of oxidation. The exposure time in the autoclave varies with the nature of the items, the size of the load, and the type of containers or wraps being sterilized.

Steam, since it is water saturation, has the disadvantages of rusting, corroding, and dulling the cutting edges of certain instruments, most particularly those made of carbon steel. Use of certain chemical additives to water, such as one percent sodium nitrite, has been advocated to prevent instrument damage in autoclaves. But such additives sometimes result in residuals on instruments; therefore, the treatment has not been widely accepted. Steam saturation also creates the need to dry the load after completion of the cycle, since packages and items must not be stored when moist. Certain plastics, rubbers, and other materials sensitive to heat and moisture cannot be sterilized in a steam autoclave without damage.

As with dry heat, autoclaves have a tendency to stratify and to trap air in pockets, thereby precluding sterilization. It is necessary, therefore, in order to minimize the occurrence of steam stratification and air pockets, to evacuate most of the air from the autoclave chamber prior to admitting the water or pre-heated steam. Pre-evacuation is accomplished in table-top autoclaves through a gravity air-displacement valve, which acts to maintain the proper pressure-temperature relationship. It is very important to compare pressures and temperatures and to make certain the correct relationships are attained and maintained. It is also important to use only deionized water in autoclaves, because prolonged use of tap water, which usually contains minerals, may damage the unit.

As previously mentioned, the American Dental Association has guidelines for acceptance of autoclaves under the ADA Acceptance Program.[5] Following are some of the more important excerpts from these guidelines:

> *The sterilizer shall be listed by the Underwriters Laboratories, Incorporated.*
>
> *The sterilizing pressure vessels shall meet the requirements of the ASME Boiler and Pressure Vessel Code.*
>
> *All instructions, directions, and information will be written in language easily understood by laypersons operating the sterilizer.*
>
> *A manual will be provided with illustrated instructions to explain proper operation and loading of the sterilizer.*
>
> *The autoclave sterilizer will be evaluated for its publicized performance and its ability to sterilize.*
>
> *The sterilizer must be capable of destroying bacterial spores.*

Many of these same requirements also apply to the chemical vapor sterilization method. It is the intention of the ADA to develop guidelines for the acceptance of all methods of sterilization that are not presently covered under the Acceptance Program.

Chemical Vapor Sterilization

The chemical vapor sterilization process was patented in 1928 by Dr. George Hollenback,[6] and a functional sterilizer came into use in dentistry following World War II. The system depends on heat, water, and chemical synergism for efficacy. The solution used in the system contains specific amounts of alcohols, acetone, ketone, formaldehyde, and water. The water content is kept below the approximate fifteen percent threshold level where rust, corrosion, and dullness of metals occur. Thus the formulation, when heated to 270 °F (131 °C) and 20 p.s.i. pressure, results in an unsaturated sterilization vapor which does not damage metal surfaces.[7][8]

(See Figures 40 and 41.) Since the chemical vapors contain much less water than the steam in autoclaves, penetration of absorbent materials, such as textiles, is slower.

The solution used in the sterilizer produces a chemical odor when heated, and although the vapors are not harmful, adequate ventilation must be provided, especially when multiple sterilizers are used in a small area. The manufacturer of the chemical vapor sterilizer also offers a filtration unit which effectively removes most of the chemical odor upon completion of the cycle. This option should be considered if the sterilizer is to be used in areas with minimal ventilation.

The fact that the chemical vapor sterilizer does not harm metals is important because the system offers faster instrument turn-around time than does dry heat and also offers more protection to certain carbon steel instruments, such as burs, knives, and other such cutting instruments, than that offered in steam autoclaves. (See Figures 40 and 41.) Many "sharp" instruments are made of carbon steel, and dentists may neglect to sterilize carbon steel because they are aware that autoclaves may damage such instruments.

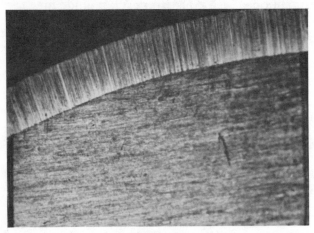

FIGURE 40
Scalpel sterilized four times in a chemical vapor sterilizer.

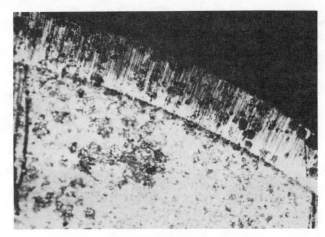

FIGURE 41
Scalpel sterilized four times in an autoclave.

The chemical vapor sterilizer offers a practical way of sterilizing instruments, items made of metal, and many other items, thereby eliminating many of the dangers of cross-contamination possible with the use of instruments which may have been only disinfected.

A recently study by Loma Linda University[9] showed that sixty-eight percent of the dental burs and forty-six percent of the basic operative instruments used in the private offices studied were not sterilized, but were merely disinfected. Additionally, a 1979 study[10] of fifty orthodontic offices concluded that forty-seven of fifty of the offices studied relied TOTALLY on cold disinfection solution for instrument treatment. To compound the problem, forty-nine of the fifty offices used quaternary ammoniums, which have been shown, as early as 1975, to be unacceptable for instrument disinfection. Imagine the possibilities for cross-contamination in such offices. Orthodontic patients often have a high degree of exposure because of their youth and their increased susceptibility to certain disorders such as infectious mononucleosis.

In summary, of the four generally accepted methods of dental sterilization, dry heat should be considered when low cost is a primary concern. The trade-off for lower cost is a substantially longer sterilization time. Liquid glutaraldehydes should be considered mainly as an adjunct to heat sterilization for sterilizing heat-sensitive items. Autoclaves should be considered where textile and solution sterilization are important concerns. Chemical vapor sterilizers should be considered where turn-around time and protection of instruments are important. All methods of sterilization fill a need when used as designed. No single method is perfect, and since there is no all purpose sterilizer, many busy offices may need several methods to satisfy all sterility needs. One or more heat systems, together with limited use of glutaraldehydes, may be necessary to complete the sterility assurance armamentarium.

For those persons wishing additional information on sterilizers, the American Dental Association has some excellent publications, including *Accepted Dental Therapeutics; Dentist's Desk Reference: Materials, Instruments and Equipment;* ADA Council reports; and the ADA Sterilization Chart.

Sterilizer Instructions

After purchasing a sterilizer, it is very important that the buyer compare the manufacturer's instructions against published guidelines, particularly regarding sterility times, pressures, and temperature. When the manufacturer's instructions vary from well-established guidelines, the guidelines should be followed. Occasionally, competitive pressure may make a manufacturer overzealous in claims which are not supported by scientific evidence. For example, some dry heat manufacturers recommend sterilization times which are substantially shorter than well-accepted guidelines, and their claims are not supported with adequate independent scientific claims. Good sources for comparing a manufacturer's claims are *Accepted Dental Therapeutics* and *Dentist's Desk Reference: Materials, Instruments and Equipment,* both published by the American Dental Association, *The U.S. Pharmacopoeia,* and *Sterilization, Disinfection and Preservation* by S.S. Block.[11]

Once the instructions for use are understood, they should be permanently attached to the sterilizer as a reminder to operators. The instructions should also include directions for cleaning, maintenance, and biological monitoring.

Sterilizer Indicators and Monitors

Selecting the correct sterilizer does not guarantee that dependably repetitive sterilization will be accomplished with the unit. The sterilizer must function correctly and the operator of the unit must use it properly. Sterilizers occasionally fail mechanically, and periodic changes of operators are unavoidable. When operators change, the new operator may not receive full and correct training and, therefore, may not fully comprehend the functions of the sterilizer. Every new operator should be required to review the manufacturer's instructions and should be required to read published guidelines for the sterilizer being used. IT IS ALSO VERY IMPORTANT THAT THE DENTIST SUPERVISE TRAINING OF NEW INFECTION CONTROL PERSONNEL. It is very easy to ask the departing operator to train the replacement, but a departing employee no longer has a vested interest in the practice and may not take the time necessary to thoroughly train the replacement in all aspects of infection control. It is equally important that the dentist keep abreast of the latest procedures.

Even with efficient operators, it is very important that a monitoring system be utilized to check for proper mechanical function and correct operator use of the sterilizer. Utilization of process indicators and biological monitors is a valuable aid in assuring effective sterilization.

Process Indicators

The two most commonly used indicators for checking sterility procedures are process indicators and biological monitors. Process indicators, sometimes called chemical indicators, are usually composed of an ink compound on paper, tape, or cardboard. The ink changes color with heat and/or steam or chemical vapors, thereby "indicating" that the load has been "processed." A few specialized process indicators are made of wax or liquid sealed in vials or plastic tubes.

Some process indicators are designed only for use in a particular sterilization method and may not be used in other methods. Manufacturer's instructions should be followed closely to prevent false indications from use of inappropriate indicators.

PROCESS INDICATORS DO NOT PROVE STERILIZATION. They rely on color change to verify only that the items being processed have been subjected to certain processing conditions. The main function of a process indicator is to prevent the inadvertent operator error of not cycling a load through the sterilizer.

Busy offices often have several persons working in the instrument recirculation center, and the possibility of error always exists. A quick look to confirm that the process indicator has changed color helps to minimize error. An illustration of the process indicator, before and after use, should be posted near the sterilizer for operators to compare as necessary.

A more sophisticated process indicator, called a control indicator, certified indicator, or an integrator, more closely matches the ink color change to prescribed sterility times, temperatures, and pressures. The control indicator system includes a sterilized "model" strip for comparing the color change obtained during the cycle to the control "model." The color change is catalyzed by temperature, time, and sometimes steam or chemical vapor pressure. If the sterilized processed indicator matches the control, the prescribed sterilization parameters have been met. Control indicators are not as assuring as the use of a biological monitor. No chemical process can provide the same dependability as that provided by the actual killing of known numbers of resistant spores.

Regardless of the type of indicator chosen for use in the office, at least one process indicator should be cycled with every sterilization load, and the results should be recorded and kept in a sterility assurance file. (See Figure 44 for examples of process indicators.)

Biological Monitors

Biological monitors are small strips of special paper to which a precise number of live, resistant spores has been applied. Each strip is

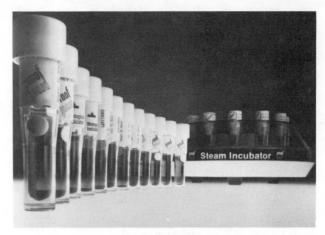

FIGURE 42
One type of self-contained biological monitor.

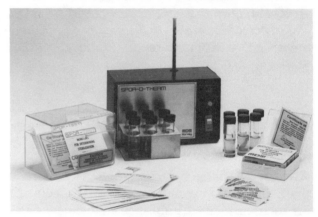

FIGURE 43
Various configurations of biological monitors.

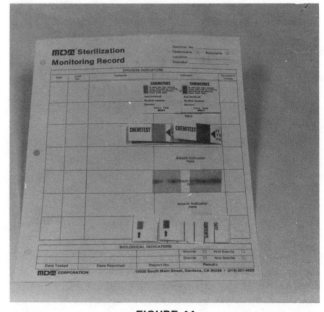

FIGURE 44
Quality Assurance Sterility Record Sheet with processed indicators.

packaged in a protective envelope or tube, which can be penetrated by steam or vapors, but which is not penetrable by the microorganisms. Therefore, the strips are safe for handling by operators.

BIOLOGICAL MONITORS ARE DESIGNED TO PROVE STERILIZATION through the process of completely killing known quantities of highly resistant spores. If the spores are killed, less resistant microbes are killed even more rapidly, and sterility is achieved.

Certain species of spores are more resistant to kill in certain methods of sterilization. *Bacillus stearothermophilus* resists kill in autoclaves and in chemical vapor sterilizers and is, therefore, the species of choice for testing those systems. *Bacillus subtilis* resists kill in dry heat sterilizers and is, therefore, the species of choice for testing that system. Unfortunately, there is no practical test for monitoring glutaraldehydes. Only the recommended species of spores should be used for monitoring the sterilization method being tested, and the monitors should not be used beyond the date specified on the package, since spores become less resistant as they age. Manufacturer's instructions for storing monitors should be followed closely because excessive heat may shorten the resistance life of the spores.

Biological monitors should be used at least once each month in each sterilizer in private offices and at least once each week in each sterilizer in busy clinics, institutions, or hospitals.[12] The American Dental Association, Veteran's Administration, Defense Medical Materiel Board, the Joint Commission for Accreditation of Hospitals, and most institutions require biological monitoring on a weekly basis.

Biological monitors should be placed in the sterilizer where sterilization may be most difficult, such as inside trays and bags, or between layers of textiles or instruments. When spores are sterilized in hard to reach parts of the sterilizer, sterility is assured in other areas.

Following cycling, each biological strip must be cultured for seventy-two hours before the results of the testing are final. Culturing may be done by a commercial laboratory or by a person in the dental office. The technique of microbiological culturing is not difficult to learn and consists of aseptically transferring the sterilized strips from the glassine envelopes to tubes of culture media. The strips are then incubated at 56 or 37 degrees centigrade, depending on the species of spores. Color-coded media are available for easily interpreting results. The growth of the spores causes a chemical reaction which changes the color of the media. Reading is quick and easy. An unsterilized control must be cultured at the same time to prove that the spores and culture media are suitable. Three days is a long time to wait for results, but there is no way to shorten the culture growth process. Sterility failures often show in less than seventy-two hours and corrective action may be taken immediately, but final reading must wait for seventy-two hours.

Two companies offer biological monitors which are pre-packaged with the biological strip separated from culture media in a single vial. The entire unit is sterilized and then, following sterilization, the operator breaks the inside culture container to mix the culture media and strip aseptically in the outer vial. Each company supplies an incubator for culturing its own vials in the office. One of the manufacturers instructs the user not to culture the strips for more than forty-eight hours. This test is questionable because some microbes, which have only been "injured" in the sterilizer, may not show growth until after forty-eight hours. These in-office, self-contained tests are attractive because of the simplicity of use and the ease of culturing and reading. As would be expected, the cost is somewhat higher than that of other in-office systems.

There are also spore testing products in other configurations. Complete services are available from commercial concerns and from at least one dental school which include the spore packages, instructions, return packaging, culturing, reading, and written reporting of results. Following cycling, the packages may be returned to the manufacturer or to another laboratory, who then will culture the strips, read the results, and issue a certifying report. For offices with multiple sterilizers, complete in-office systems are available with bulk packages of spore strips, culture media, and a small incubator. Staff can be taught easily to process the strips. Use of this type of in-office system is less expensive than the self-contained tests.

The results of process indicators and biological monitors should be recorded and kept as a part of a complete sterility assurance program. Pre-printed forms are available which take only a few minutes each day to complete. (See Figure 44.) This proof of sterility is potentially valuable in protecting dental staff from liability in case of a malpractice suit.

References and Suggested Readings

1. ADA Council on Dental Therapeutics. "Quaternary Ammonium Compounds Not Acceptable for Disinfection of Instruments and Environmental Surfaces." JADA 97(5):855, 1978.

2. Kolstad Chemiclave and Glutaraldehyde Sterilization. Unpublished Report, Baylor Univ, 1982.

3. Whitacre, R.J., et al., eds. DENTAL ASEPSIS. Stoma Press, Inc. Seattle or J. Crawford, Univ of NC Dent Sch, Chapel Hill, 1979.

4. Metchnikoff, E. THE FOUNDER OF MODERN MEDICINE (Pasteur, Koch, Lister), (New York: Walden Publication, 1939).

5. Runnells, R.R. INFECTION CONTROL IN THE WET FINGER ENVIRONMENT (Publishers Press, N. Salt Lake, UT, 1984).

6. Hollenback, G.M. *Patent Number 1663841*, March 27, 1928.

7. Haberman, S. "Some Comparative Studies Between a Chemical Vapor Sterilizer and a Conventional Steam Autoclave on Various Bacteria and Viruses," May, 1962, Jnl So Cal St Dent Assn, XXX:5:163-172.

8. Lyon, T.C. and Devine, M.J. "Evaluation of a New Model Vapor Pressure Sterilizer," Feb, 1974, Jnl of Dent Res, 53:634.

9. Rathbun, G. "Is There Life After Sterilization?" Unpublished report, 1983, Loma Linda Univ, Dept of Dent Hyg.

10. Matlack, R.E. "Instrument Sterilization in Orthodontic Offices," July, 1979, The Ang Ortho, 49:3:205-211.

11. Block, S.S. *Sterilization, Disinfection and Preservation.* Second Edition (Philadelphia: Lea and Febiger, 1977).

12. Runnells, R.R. and Schmoegner, J.S. "The Need to Monitor Use and Function of Sterilizers," Oct, 1980, Dent Surv, 56:10:20-24.

Chapter Nine
REVIEW EXERCISES

Date _____Name_____

Circle the letters of the terms which most closely approximate the answers. There may be one or more than one correct answer. If you circle D, indicate the other answer or answers, if known.

1. Choosing the most practical sterilizer is important because:

   A. it is important not to waste money

   B. sterilization must be fast

   C. the sterilizer is the heart of infection control

   D. other_____

2. The best "cold sterilizing" solution is:

   A. inexpensive

   B. quaternary ammonium

   C. simple boiling water

   D. other_____

3. Almost all "cold sterilizing solutions" used in dentistry are:

   A. disinfectants

   B. chemical compounds

   C. effective

   D. other_____

4. Liquid disinfectants should be used mostly:

   A. when speed is important

   B. for most expensive instruments

   C. for heat sensitive items

   D. other_____

5. The Environmental Protection Agency regulates:

   A. autoclaves

   B. dry heat sterilizers

   C. chemical vapor sterilizers

   D. other_____

6. The American Dental Association presently studies and accepts the following system:

   A. autoclaves   B. glutaraldehydes   C. chemical vapor sterilizers

   D. other_____

7. Some sterilizers sold in the United States are:

   A. regulated   B. impractical for office use   C. not regulated

   D. other_____

8. When selecting a sterilizer one should:

   A. consult dental suppliers   B. study published sterility   C. consult the local hospital
                                        guidelines

   D. other_____

9. Of the methods of sterilization available in the United States:

   A. all are practical for   B. four are practical for   C. two are practical for
      dentistry   dentistry   dentistry

   D. other_____

10. Sterilization parameters for autoclaves include:

    A. 250-275 degrees F.   B. one hour cycle   C. automatic drying cycle
       temperature

    D. other_____

11. One sterilization cycle for dry heat includes:

    A. 20-minute cycle   B. 320 degrees F. temperature   C. 40-minute cycle

    D. other_____

12. Sterilization parameters for chemical vapor sterilizers includes:

    A. 20-minute cycle   B. 270 degrees F. temperature   C. 40-minute cycle

    D. other_____

13. Sterilization parameters for liquid glutaraldehydes includes:

A. room temperature   B. two-hour cycle   C. 6¾-10 hour cycle

D. other_____

14. A potentially most expensive method of sterilization is:

A. dry heat   B. one that does not sterilize   C. steam autoclave

D. other_____

15. The item(s) best suited for sterilization in the autoclave is/are:

A. instruments   B. solutions   C. textiles

D. other_____

16. The item(s) best suited for sterilization in the chemical vapor sterilizer is/are:

A. instruments   B. glassware and dry   C. textiles
                            chemicals

D. other_____

17. The item(s) best suited for sterilization in the dry heat sterilizer is/are:

A. instruments   B. glassware and dry   C. certain plastics
                            chemicals

D. other_____

18. The item(s) best suited for sterilization in liquid glutaraldehyde is/are:

A. instruments   B. certain plastics   C. low-temperature items

D. other_____

19. The most practical sterilizer(s) for use in busy dental offices is/are:

A. autoclave   B. chemical vapor sterilizer   C. dry heat

D. other_____

20. To satisfy most sterilization needs, busy dental practices may require:

A. a very large sterilizer   B. an expensive sterilizer   C. several different sterilizers

D. other_____

21. The oldest and best known method of sterilization is:

A. dry heat   B. autoclave   C. chemical vapor sterilizer

D. other_____

22. Dry heat is an acceptable method of sterilization for non-high-heat sensitive instruments when:

A. glutaraldehyde is not available   B. fast turn-around is not necessary   C. fast turn-around is necessary

D. other_____

23. The autoclave is a primary method of sterilization for textiles because of:

A. faster penetration   B. higher temperatures   C. shorter cycle

D. other_____

24. The chemical vapor sterilizer is a primary method of sterilization for instruments because of:

A. lower temperatures   B. less adverse effect on certain metals   C. fast turn-around

D. other_____

25. The autoclave and the dry heat sterilizer are similar in that they:

A. are made of metal   B. utilize a similar pressure chamber   C. have a tendency to stratify or trap air

D. other_____

26. For fast turn-around, carbon steel instruments should be sterilized in:

A. liquid glutaraldehyde   B. chemical vapor sterilizer   C. autoclave

D. other_____

27. The least sterilized instrument in many offices is the:

   A. periodontal knife   B. dental bur   C. curette

   D. other_____

28. Liquid glutaraldehydes should be used as:

   A. the main method of   B. a better disinfectant   C. an adjunct to a heat
      sterilization in new offices   sterilizer

   D. other_____

29. Liquid glutaraldehydes are:

   A. all the same   B. available in several forms   C. only disinfectants

   D. other_____

30. Sterilizer manufacturer's instructions for use should be:

   A. supported by   B. checked against published   C. available by phone
      independent studies   guidelines

   D. other_____

31. A good source for checking some sterilizer manufacturers' claims is:

   A. *Consumer Report*   B. *Accepted Dental*   C. Environment Protection
                                 Therapeutics   Agency *Guidelines*

   D. other_____

32. Sterilizer instructions should be:

   A. read and kept   B. memorized and filed for   C. permanently affixed to the
                                 review   sterilizer

   D. other_____

33. Choosing a specific sterilizer(s) guarantees:

   A. sterility when the   B. nothing   C. disinfection at the very least
      unit is used correctly

   D. other_____

34. Use of process indicators and biological monitors:

A. helps assure effective
   sterilization

B. helps protect against
   malpractice suits

C. is expensive

D. other_____

35. Process indicators:

A. prove sterilization

B. rely on chemical ink
   color change

C. contain live spores

D. other_____

36. The main function(s) of process indicators is/are:

A. to show that loads
   have been processed

B. to check on mechanical
   function of the sterilizer

C. to check on operator
   procedures

D. other_____

37. A control process indicator is:

A. a certified indicator

B. a biological monitor

C. to check on the quality of
   other indicators

D. other_____

38. Biological monitors are:

A. proof of sterility

B. metal strips covered with
   live spores

C. badges worn during sterility
   exposure

D. other_____

39. Biological monitors must be:

A. used in every
   sterility load

B. incubated for 24 hours

C. incubated for 72 hours

D. other_____

40. Biological monitors can be:

A. used to prove sterility in all sterilization methods

B. handled safely in packages

C. dangerous even when handled correctly

D. other_____

41. Biological monitors should be placed in:

A. most difficult to sterilize areas in chamber

B. small glassine envelopes

C. metal culture tubes

D. other_____

42. The spore species of choice for monitoring an autoclave is:

A. *Bacillus subtilis*

B. *Clostridium sporogenes*

C. *Bacillus stearothermophilus*

D. other_____

43. The spore species of choice for monitoring a chemical vapor sterilizer is:

A. *Bacillus subtilis*

B. *Clostridium sporogenes*

C. *Bacillus stearothermophilus*

D. other_____

44. The spore species of choice for monitoring a dry heat sterilizer is:

A. *Bacillus subtilis*

B. *Clostridium sporogenes*

C. *Bacillus stearothermophilus*

D. other_____

45. The spore species of choice for monitoring liquid glutaraldehydes sterilant is:

A. *Bacillus subtilis*

B. *Clostridium sporogenes*

C. *Bacillus stearothermophilus*

D. other_____

46. The least expensive way to use biological monitors is:

A. to use only one

B. to use in-office system

C. to use less often

D. other_____

47. Process indicators and biological monitors should both be:

A. used every day

B. used weekly or monthly depending on how busy the practice

C. used and results recorded and kept

D. other_____

NOTE: Answers to review exercises appear in the back of this book.

The Instrument Recirculation Center

ABSTRACT: The instrument recirculation center is as important as any dental patient treatment area. The center is not a source of direct income to the dentist, but it makes a substantial contribution to profit by stimulating an increase in personnel efficiency and by assisting in the prevention of infective cross-contamination.

Once the dentist and staff have selected the various components of a sterility assurance program, those components should be organized for the most effective use in an instrument recirculation center. The instrument recirculation center serves a number of needs:

1. Organization of sterility components, such as cleaner, sterilizer(s), packaging material, etc.

2. Control of microbial count.

3. Procedural flow.

4. Separation of contaminated objects from sterile or clean objects.

5. Obscuring of "unsightly" objects from patient view.

6. Storage of sterile items until needed.

New Construction

In new construction, the instrument recirculation center should be designed to assure efficient instrument flow, to separate the cleaning area from the sterilizing area, to offer maximum protection of stored instruments, to provide an air evacuation system for reducing a microbial count, and to incorporate other proven procedures which may have been originated by the infection control personnel of the office.

The instrument recirculation center should be constructed of smooth, non-porous materials. Metal or formica are best because they have fewer cracks, crevices, and rough surfaces where microbes may "hide," and because they are easier to clean and disinfect than are rough, irregular surfaces. Internal corners and joints should be coved to minimize crevices where microbes may accumulate and multiply. Shelves and drawers in frequently used cabinets should be removable for ease of cleaning and disinfection. This is especially necessary for storage areas and drawers in which sterilized packages will be kept.

It is very desirable to have a low volume, continuous-flow air evacuation system pulling air upward from the work areas. The upward movement of air will help reduce the number of airborne microbes in the center. The evacuated air should be pulled through a microbial filter, and the filter should be replaced frequently, at least monthly in busy offices. It is also desirable to vent potentially offensive odors or vapors generated by autoclaves and chemical vapor sterilizers to the outside. When the instrument recirculation center is planned, vents or spaces should be left between and behind cabinets to assure movement of the air through the evacuation system. Cabinets and drawers should be tightly closed to prevent the air movement from carrying airborne microorganisms into the storage areas.

Existing Offices

In existing offices, where new construction or remodeling is not possible, every effort should be made to use existing space most efficiently. Wherever possible, instrument recirculation should be kept away from treatment areas and from the laboratory. Occasional compromise may be provided by a partial partition or divider for separation of the functions. In smaller spaces, separation of the various steps of instrument processing may not be possible. Even in such cases, every effort should be made to effectively separate the handling and cleaning of contaminated instruments from the packaging, sterilization, and storage. It may require ingenuity on the part of infection control personnel, but the recirculation functions can usually be effectively accomplished.

Instrument Flow

Following is a diagram of the functions to be performed in an instrument recirculation center and the preferred order of flow for maximal control and efficiency:

These functions may be organized in a single wall eight to ten feet in length (see Figure 45), or they may be separated into two walls with each section approximately eight to ten feet in length (see Figure 46). In either case, the functions and flow should remain the same. Capacity, surface area, and ease of operator movement are the main variables.

In the single wall, it is preferable to build the sterilizer into the cabinetry to conserve surface space (see Figure 45). If desired, the sterilizer(s) may be surface mounted in the double wall center. Use of the double wall is necessary if two or more sterilizers are to be utilized.

The most efficient layout of the wall will allow access (either by way of a pass-through window or cabinets which open on both sides) to the sterile instrument storage from both the recirculation center and the patient treatment area. A pass-through window on the contaminated side is not indicated because cleaning procedures in the recirculation center may allow microbes to enter in the patient treatment area through the opening.

The following two figures suggest an efficient layout of a single and double wall instrument recirculation center.

Single Wall Instrument Recirculation Center

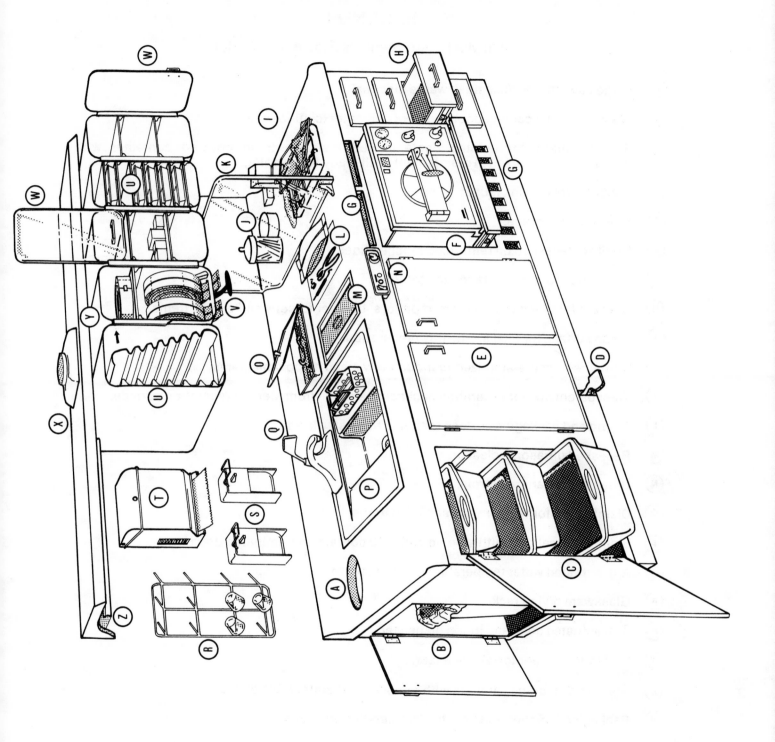

FIGURE 45

LEGEND I

Single Wall Instrument Recirculation Center

(A) Large capacity, surface flush waste disposal.

(B) Waste disposal cabinet door in rear of cabinetry to utilize space.

(C) Storage space for holding contaminated instruments in covered container with instruments immersed in disinfectant until ready for cleaning.

(D) Foot control for sink faucet.

(E) Bulk supply storage.

(F) Sterilizer recessed on reinforced mobile glides.

(G) Ventilation for air circulation to sterilizer.

(H) Drawers for process indicators, monitors, transfer forceps and similar items.

(I) Clean surface for final sterile tray preparation.

(J) Containers for pre-sterilized or industrially clean disposable items.

(K) Transparent divider separating packaging surface from sterile preparation surface.

(L) Drying and packaging surface for items to be sterilized.

(M) Recessed ultrasonic cleaner.

(N) Ultrasonic cleaner controls.

(O) Disinfectant for temperature sensitive items.

(P) Stainless steel sink with sloping drains to contain contaminated drain water.

(Q) Arm actuated water temperature mixture control.

(R) Glassware drying rack.

(S) Arm actuated soap and lotion dispenser.

(T) "No touch" paper towel dispenser.

(U) Sterile tray storage cabinets with removable, disinfectable slides.

(V) Packaging supplies and "cut to size" see-through bags.

(W) Glass or solid doors.

(X) Low volume air evacuation system with microbial filter.

(Y) Air movement space between cabinets.

(Z) Light.

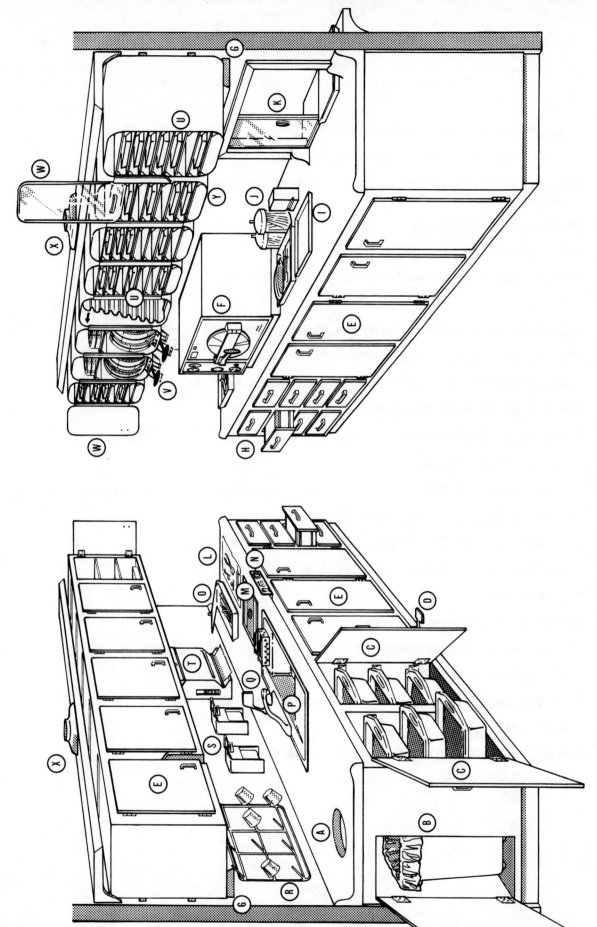

Double Wall Instrument Recirculation center

FIGURE 46

LEGEND II
Double Wall Instrument Recirculation Center

(A) Large capacity, surface flush waste disposal.

(B) Waste disposal cabinet door in rear of cabinetry to utilize space.

(C) Storage space for holding contaminated instruments in covered container immersed in disinfectant until ready for cleaning.

(D) Foot control for sink faucet.

(E) Bulk supply storage.

(F) Sterilizer, cabinet top or recessed on reinforced mobile glides.

(G) Lights.

(H) Drawers for process indicators, monitors, transfer forceps, and similar items.

(I) Clean surface for final sterile tray preparation.

(J) Containers for pre-sterilized or industrially clean disposable items.

(K) Pass-through window to treatment area.

(L) Drying surface for items to be sterilized.

(M) Recessed ultrasonic cleaner.

(N) Ultrasonic cleaner controls.

(O) Disinfectant for temperature sensitive items.

(P) Stainless steel sink with sloping drain to contain contaminated drain water.

(Q) Arm actuated water temperature mixture control.

(R) Glassware drying rack.

(S) Arm actuated soap and lotion dispenser.

(T) "No touch" paper towel dispenser.

(U) Sterile tray storage cabinets with removable, disinfectable slides.

(V) Packaging supplies and "cut to size" see-through bags.

(W) Glass or solid doors.

(X) Low volume air evacuation system with microbial filter.

(Y) Air movement space between cabinets.

Chapter Ten
REVIEW EXERCISES

Date _____ Name_____

Circle the letters of the terms which most closely approximate the answers. There may be one or more than one correct answer. If you circle D, indicate the other answer or answers, if known.

1. The most important function of the instrument recirculation center is to:

    A. assure efficient   B. keep instruments orderly   C. provide for instrument
       instrument flow   storage

    D. other_____

2. Instrument recirculation centers preferably should be constructed of:

    A. aesthetically pleasing   B. all metal   C. metal and formica
       wood

    D. other_____

3. Effective instrument recirculation may be utilized in:

    A. new offices   B. existing offices   C. busy clinics

    D. other_____

4. Dental sink faucets should be:

    A. hand operated   B. forearm operated   C. electric eye operated

    D. other_____

5. All dental dispensers should be:

    A. on the counter top   B. metal   C. wall hung

    D. other_____

6. Waste receptacles should be:

    A. large   B. metal   C. hidden

    D. other_____

NOTE: Answers to review exercises are in the back of this book.

Instrument Recirculation

ABSTRACT: If only one infection control emphasis could be practiced, the cleaning, packaging, sterilization, and recirculation of instruments would be that emphasis.

The procedures of instrument recirculation are not difficult, but they do require observance of certain basic procedures.

The practice of effective procedures and the use of high quality sterilization equipment and supplies for recirculation of instruments offer the greatest single opportunity for controlling cross-contamination in an infection control program. Most instruments are used directly in the mouth, contacting saliva and blood, and are thereby exposed to the highest concentration of potential pathogens. As a result, there is a great threat to patients through the possible cutting or "invading" of oral mucosa with instruments. It is nearly impossible to treat a patient without invading the mucosa with a bur, forceps, elevator, retainer, rubber dam clamp, wedge, or any of the other diverse instruments or devices used in dental procedures. Every time the mucosa is broken, the patient is potentially exposed to infection. The threat is not only to patients. Every time a sharp instrument or device is handled by dental personnel, the same threat of infection is present through the danger of cuts, nicks, or abrasions to fingers or hands.

Many studies have shown that most personnel working in or near the mouth frequently cut or nick their fingers. Handling explorers, changing burs, pressing separators and wedges to place, handling suture needles, seating orthodontic bands, rotating reamers and files, scrubbing instruments, and the multitude of other "hand-finger procedures" almost guarantee skin punctures and abrasions. Once the skin is broken, the resulting wound is susceptible to bacterial invasion for hours or even days.

It cannot be emphasized too strongly that EVERYTHING THAT CAN BE STERILIZED MUST BE STERILIZED. Furthermore, sterilized instruments and items must be protected from recontamination until ready for use.

A FIFTH GOAL OF INFECTION CONTROL IS THAT ALL PROCEDURES USED IN THE INSTRUMENT RECIRCULATION CENTER MUST BE REPETITIVE, EFFICIENT, AND COMPLETE.

Instrument recirculation involves the handling and cleaning, the packaging and sterilizing, and the storing and preparation of all instruments used in the dental treatment areas. All of these steps must be accomplished without the exposure of patients or staff to cross-contamination.

143

These rules are inviolate:

1. Place all used instruments in a disinfecting solution until cleaning can be accomplished.

2. After the patient leaves, never handle contaminated instruments without using latex utility gloves. (See Figure 48.)

3. Pre-package all instruments for sterilization, with the possible exception of a few that will be immediately re-used the same day.

4. Sterilize EVERYTHING which can be sterilized. Only when absolutely necessary consider liquid disinfectants as a compromise to be used in the place of sterilization.

5. Use a proven method of sterilization which will most closely satisfy office needs.

6. Never place unpackaged, sterilized instruments directly on non-sterile surfaces. Always cover surfaces first with a sterile towel, paper or other protective disposable cover.

7. Routinely check, with process indicators and biological monitors, the efficiency of instrument recirculation procedures and the mechanical function of sterilizers.

8. Maintain sterilization records in a sterility assurance file.

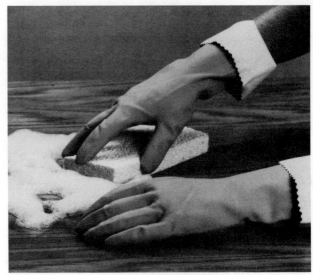

FIGURE 48
One type of protective gloves.

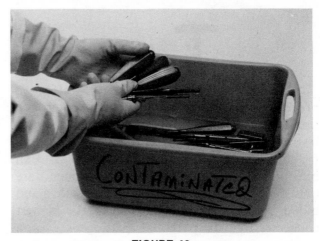

FIGURE 49
Handling contaminated instruments in a contaminated container.

Handling Instruments

After the patient leaves, assistants should wear heavy, utility protective rubber gloves and should immediately place contaminated instruments in a covered container partially filled with liquid disinfectant. In some offices, a tray partially filled with disinfectant is placed near treatment personnel at the beginning of patient treatment. Used instruments are immediately placed in the liquid after the last use. This procedure is especially useful during long operative procedures where blood and serum may dry on instruments during the extended treatment.

Keeping the instruments covered with a liquid until cleaning will prevent drying of blood and

serum on the instruments and will make cleaning easier and more effective. Contaminated, one-time use materials, disposable items, and other treatment debris should be placed in a plastic bag to be disposed of, preferably by incineration, at the end of each day. Needles and surgical blades should be disposed of separately in a puncture proof, secure container, as previously described.

Instruments should be stored in the liquid disinfectant until ready for cleaning, then rinsed under hot running water. Hot water assures the most efficient removal of gross debris. If a large amount of blood is present, rinse with cool water, then hot water. An ultrasonic cleaner should be used for instrument cleaning since the use of such a cleaner has been reported to be up to sixteen times more efficient than hand scrubbing.[1] Ultrasonic cleaning is also safer because hand scrubbing exposes personnel to cuts and finger nicks, even through utility gloves. A lid should always be used to cover the ultrasonic cleaner when in use, and the solution should be changed frequently, as often as daily in areas of high usage. Use of an uncovered cleaner may result in contaminated aerosol splash, since the ultrasonic action causes an "implosion of bubbles" with a resultant splashing and vaporizing of the solution.

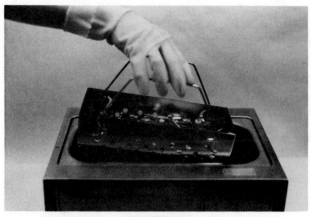

FIGURE 50
Ultrasonically cleaning instruments.

Efficiency of ultrasonic cleaning action tends to degrade with use. It is desirable to check the action periodically to assure efficient cleaning. A simple test of cleaning action is afforded through use of a small piece of regular weight aluminum foil. The foil should be partially immersed vertically into fresh solution with the cleaner functioning. After 20 seconds immersion, the foil should show small pinholes in the immersed section. If not, the cleaner may be in need of repair or replacement.

An ultrasonic cleaner is not a sterilizer. Although some microorganisms may be destroyed in a heated solution, many microbes survive the action and the solution becomes increasingly contaminated as more instruments

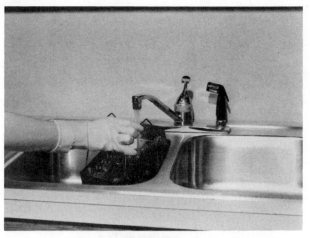

FIGURE 51
Rinsing instruments.

are cleaned. Frequent changing of the solution is an absolute necessity.

After being cleaned, the instruments should be thoroughly rinsed under cool, running water. Care should be exercised to prevent splashing of water at the sink. Most ultrasonic cleaning solutions contain some detergent, and the cool water is more effective in rinsing the soap residuals from the instruments. Instruments should be separated during rinsing to assure more effective removal of all debris and cleaning solution. Any cleaning solution left on instruments, especially in the chemical vapor sterilizer, may contribute to residual stains.

The instruments may then be placed on a clean, dry towel and rolled or patted with a second towel until most of the water is removed. Heavy gloves should be used to protect hands during patting. Leaving water on the instruments can lead to increased instrument spotting in autoclaves and to rusting, dulling, and corrosion in chemical vapor and dry heat sterilizers.

As an alternative to pat-drying, instruments may be placed in alcohol or the residual solution of the chemical vapor sterilizer. Immersion of instruments in an alcohol solution before sterilizing them removes water residue without the necessity of handling the instruments. As previously stated, to minimize the possibility of hand cuts or nicks which may lead to personnel infection, one should not handle instruments more than necessary.

145

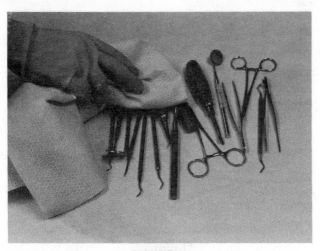

FIGURE 52
Pat drying instruments with gloved hands.

Packaging

Instruments are normally stored open-unpackaged or packaged. Historically, dentists have stored their instruments open-unpackaged in drawers on glass trays, and many dental schools will continue to allow this type of storage in portable student cabinets. The advantages of unpackaged storage are quick availability of instruments, simplicity of handling, and low cost. The problem with unpackaged storage is that it is impossible to prevent instrument re-contamination. REMOVING, USING, AND STERILIZING INSTRUMENTS AND THEN REPLACING THEM IN AN ALREADY CONTAMINATED DRAWER DEFEATS THE BASIC PRINCIPLES OF INFECTION CONTROL.

As dental packaging has evolved, especially with the introduction of covered set-up trays and sterilization bags, the storage of sterilized instruments in an aseptic environment has become fast, easy, practical, and economical.

Ideally, instruments should not be used which have not been pre-packaged in sterile containers, but it is also recognized that an infection control program must be as practical as possible to satisfy most needs. Because some offices cannot or will not adopt a complete pre-packaged storage program, the following procedure, admittedly a compromise, will assure improvement over historical instrument-storage methods.

A dentist or hygienist sometimes desires to store frequently-used instruments, such as mouth mirrors, explorers, and cotton pliers, open-unpackaged. These instruments should be sterilized and placed only in trays which are lined with disposable paper liners and on holders in the trays which are frequently sterilized or disinfected. (See Figure 53.)

The instruments in the lined trays should be widely separated on the holders so that adjacent instruments are not touched and contaminated when another instrument is removed. If adjacent instruments are touched and/or contaminated, they should be re-sterilized, whether or not they were used on a patient. Use of transfer forceps for removing instruments from holders helps minimize the risk of contamination.

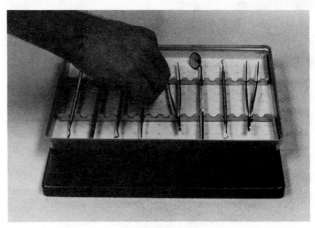

FIGURE 53
Correct way to prepare open-unpackaged tray for instrument removal.

It is highly desirable to pre-package all instruments before sterilization, even if the instruments are to be re-used again on the same day. Instruments are usually packaged, sterilized, and stored in trays, bags, or wraps.

Sterilization trays are usually available as fully-closed, perforated, and see-through. The fully-closed tray is the most dependable tray method for sterile storage of instruments, but this method has the disadvantage that the covers must be left partially open during sterilization in autoclaves and chemical vapor sterilizers to assure complete penetration by steam or chemical vapors. If the trays are not closed carefully at the end of the sterilization cycle, recontamination is possible. Fully closed trays normally require color-coding for identification of the contents to prevent the contamination of the contents when someone "peeks" into the trays.

Perforated trays are easily penetrated by steam and vapors, but the perforations must be covered with a paper liner or the contents will not remain sterile. Contamination may also occur if moisture penetrates the perforations and wets the liners. Microorganisms multiply rapidly in the presence of moisture at room temperature and become a ready source of contamination. Color coding is usually still necessary when perforated trays are used.

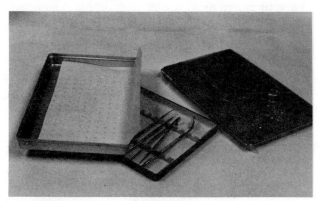

FIGURE 54
Perforated tray with liners and see-through tray.

See-through trays offer a practical method of tray storage because they allow penetration of steam or vapors without violation of the sterile contents, and the contents may be viewed without removal of the cover. A transparent nylon cover serves to protect the contents from contamination after sterilization. Since see-through trays have vents under the ends of the nylon, storage in protected areas is important to prevent contaminated air from entering the trays. See-through trays are somewhat slower to assemble than other trays, but the advantages of the system far outweigh this slight disadvantage. See-through trays are also less expensive to use than paper or see-through bags. The only cost is a disposable sheet of nylon.

A leading dental instrument manufacturer recently introduced a new storage system which allows cleaning and sterilization in the same cassette. (See Figure 55.) A similar cassette has been used successfully for a number of years at the Winston-Salem Dental Care Plan, Inc., where they recycle between 600 and 1,000 cassettes daily. The organization of the cassette assures minimal handling by personnel and maximal protection of instruments.

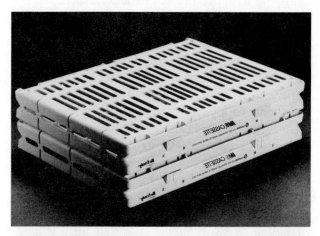

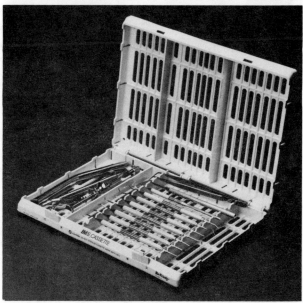

FIGURES 55 & 56
Protective cassettes for instrument circulation.

147

For those offices not wishing to use set-up trays, sterilization bags and sterilization tubing, which can be cut to the desired size and then heat-sealed, offer excellent packaging options. Bags and tubing are relatively inexpensive and are available in many sizes and configurations, including all paper or paper-plastic combinations. The clear plastic side assures easy viewing of contents. Many bags and tubings are also available with pre-printed process indicators.

When loading bags, one should not perforate the bags with sharp-pointed instruments or with the marking device used to label non-see-through paper bags. To prevent puncturing the paper, one should use a soft dull pencil rather than a hard pencil or pen. This precaution is important for a second reason when one is using a chemical vapor sterilizer, because the vapor may dissolve the ink used in pens, and the ink residue may be deposited on the chamber walls and instruments. Sharp points and edges of instruments should be covered with single layers of gauze or short pieces of small bore silicone tubing which is just long enough to securely cover the edges or the ends of the instruments. When protective tubing is used, it should be open on both ends to allow complete passage of steam or vapors. It is not advisable to protect instrument tips with cotton rolls, which may tend to inhibit sterilization.

Items which are too large to be placed in closed trays or bags should be packaged in paper or in loosely-woven muslin wraps. Paper is preferred to textile wraps for chemical vapor sterilizers because of the slower penetration of the vapors through textiles. Cloth wraps, such as those historically used by hospitals, should be avoided in both autoclaves and chemical vapor sterilizers.

Some persons trained in the use of cloth-wrapped hospital-type packs feel that cloth offers a superior method of wrapping. Cloth is re-usable; it has no "memory" and therefore can be unfolded to lie flat as a sterile working surface; and it has been used for packaging longer than paper. These are all valid considerations for used the material. There are, however, several important disadvantages to the use of cloth. Cloth is absorbent and, therefore, packs must be completely dry before being stored. The pre-

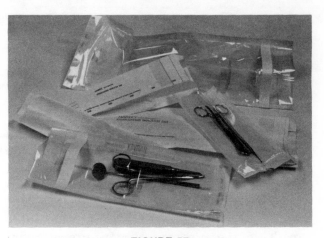

FIGURE 57
Various types of paper and paper-plastic combination bags.

sence of warm moisture creates an ideal environment for growth of microbes. If the moisture in the pack reaches the covered instruments, as it usually does in the case of an undried pack, contamination of the instruments may result. (See Table 13.) Many studies have been published on the possibility of this "wet pack syndrome."[2]

Table 13 summarizes the results of tests of bacterial penetration through muslin and six non-textile materials. The wraps were double-folded around a simulated 17-pound instrument tray and then cycled in a steam autoclave. (Reprinted from the AORN Journal, August 1983.)

Additionally, the hospital cloth-wrapping technique teaches a precise method of folding the layers of cloth. Each layer becomes more difficult for steam to penetrate and the possibility of the contents not being sterilized increases with each extra fold. Finally, studies have shown that the storage of cloth hospital packs is shorter than that of many other methods of packaging. (See Table 14.)

The use of cloth wraps has been substantially reduced in many medical disciplines, and paper wraps are becoming more popular. Because of their hospital training, oral surgeons have historically preferred the use of cloth, and in some cases they have continued to use cloth as their primary wrap. Conversion from cloth to paper should be encouraged.

TABLE 13

Bacterial penetration through the outer wrap of a double wrapped tray

Type of wrap	Percent of sites showing penetration	
	10 min	60 min
Muslin	100%	100%
Disposable wrap A	63%	86%
Disposable wrap B	40%	44%
Disposable wrap C	22%	22%
Reusable water repellent wrap	14%	22%
Polypropylene film	0%	0%
Polyethylene film	0%	0%

Chart summarizes the results of testing bacterial penetration through muslin and six non-textile materials. The wraps were double folded around an instrument tray and then cycled in a steam autoclave. Reprinted from the AORN Journal, August 1983.

TABLE 14
Safe Storage Times For Sterile Packs and Bags

Wrapping	Duration of Sterility	
	In closed cabinet	On open shelves
Single-wrapped muslin (two layers)	1 week	2 days
Double-wrapped muslin (each two layers)	7 weeks	3 weeks
Single-wrapped two-way crepe paper (single layer)	At least 8 weeks	3 weeks
Tightly woven untreated pima cotton (single layer) over single-wrapped muslin (two layers)		8 weeks
Two-way crepe paper (single layer) over single-wrapped muslin (two layers)		10 weeks
Single-wrapped muslin (two layers) sealed in 3 mil polyethylene		At least 9 months
All paper bags (tape seal)*	At least 3 months	60 days
Paper-plastic bags (tape seal)*	At least 6 months	4 months
All plastic bags (tape seal)*	1 year	6 months
*Double heat seal will increase storage times at least 30 days		

Inexpensive, one-use paper wraps are available which are also tear resistant and which allow quick penetration of steam and vapors. The disposable paper wraps are much less susceptible to "wet pack syndrome" than cloth wraps and assure longer storage life. Paper wraps should be used in the place of cloth wherever possible.

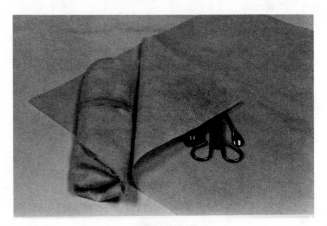
FIGURE 58
Typical disposable paper wraps.

To assure that the sterilizing process is not inhibited by the packaging, one should follow the sterilizer manufacturer's instructions concerning packaging materials. In recent years, the use of nylon tubing packaging has become popular in dentistry. Studies have shown that sterilization is sometimes inconsistent in closed nylon.[3] Penetration of steam or vapors through nylon depends on the opening of minute, penetrable holes in the nylon as the nylon is heated. The holes are then closed as the nylon cools. If the nylon is not manufactured to the precise thinness required, a sufficient number of holes do not open in the heating process; consequently, the penetration of steam or vapors is inhibited. If nylon tubing is used, certification should be obtained from the manufacturer that manufacturing tolerances are maintained to assure penetration of the heated sterilant. In the absence of this assurance, duplicate test packages, containing biological monitors, should be processed frequently, preferably daily in areas of high usage. Several test packages with biological monitors should always be processed when a new package of tubing is used.

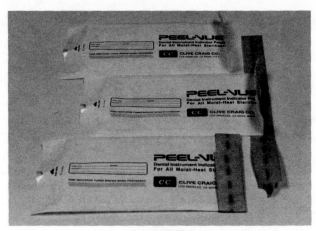
FIGURE 59
Steps in correctly sealing a bag with indicator tape.

Bags and wraps must be self-sealing or must be carefully and completely sealed with tape or heatseal. STAPLES SHOULD NOT BE USED SINCE PERFORATING WILL RESULT, AND A COMPLETE SEAL WILL NOT BE OBTAINED. When tape is used for sealing bags, the ends of the bag should be doubled back and then sealed completely with tape covering the fold and the reverse side of the bag. The closure must be fully airtight. (See Figure 59.)

Storage

Sterilized trays, bags, and wraps should be stored intact and unopened in closed, clean, dry cabinets or drawers until ready for use. The storage area should be located as far from busy traffic as possible. If located in the instrument recirculation area, the storage area should be as far from the decontamination and cleaning areas as possible. Contaminated movement of air created by busy traffic and the frequent opening and closing of cabinet doors and drawers may shorten the sterility life of the stored items. In protected areas, some see-through bags have been shown to remain sterile for at least six months.[4] Tightly-sealed all-plastic or foil bags remain sterile even longer because of the toughness and resistance of the material. Other methods of packaging have varying storage lives, with muslin or cloth wraps usually having the shortest and sealed foil bags the longest. (See

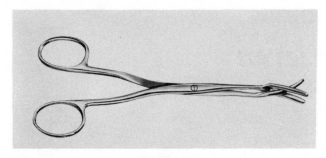

FIGURE 60
One type of sterile forceps for handling various items to prevent contamination.

Table 14.) Manufacturers' instructions concerning storage life of wraps and bags should be observed, and independent scientific studies should be made available by manufacturers to support their claims.

Table 14 summarizes the concensus of information available on safe storage times for various types of bags and wraps with varying closures. Much of the information was taken directly from guidelines developed by the Centers for Disease Control.

Tray Final Preparation

Certain dental offices may want to add disinfected or industrially clean items to the sterile set-up tray after sterilization but before use in the treatment area. For example, anesthetic cartridges, gutta percha points, paper absorbent points, rubber dams, plastic saliva ejectors, plastic HVE tips, and other similar materials may not be sterile when needed and may be available only in industrially-clean bulk containers.

It is highly desirable that non-sterile items be placed on a clean disposable barrier next to the tray in the treatment area rather than on the sterile tray. This procedure eliminates the possibility of contamination of the tray. If, however, addition of the non-sterile items to the tray is required, items should be added just before delivery of the tray to the treatment area. The earlier the items are added the greater the possibility that the tray may become contaminated.

Several pair of large transfer forceps should be sterilized with each instrument load. These forceps should be kept sterile for use in the handling of instruments and other items in the recirculation center. When one removes items such as plastic saliva ejectors from bulk packages, one should use sterile forceps to minimize the possibility of contaminating the items remaining in the package. TRANSFER FORCEPS SHOULD NOT BE STORED IN DISINFECTANT BETWEEN USES. ONLY STERILIZED FORCEPS SHOULD BE USED.

Gauze packs, cotton rolls, cotton pellets, and similar items to be added to the tray after sterilization are of special concern and should be used only when sterile. Cotton or gauge products, often used in the presence of blood, have a high possibility of contributing to cross-contamination. Such items should be added to the tray before sterilization or should be repackaged and sterilized in small bags or envelopes to be available for use during procedures. These small sterile packages eliminate the contamination possibilities always present when one uses items from non-sterile bulk packages.

References and Suggested Readings

1. Whitacre, R.J., *et al.*, eds. DENTAL ASEPSIS. Stoma Press, Inc. Seattle or J. Crawford, Univ of NC Dent Sch, Chapel Hill, 1979.

2. Karle and Ryan. "Guidelines for Evaluating Wet Packs." Assn of Oper Rm Nur Jnl, 38:2, 244-256, Aug, 1983.

3. Runnells, R.R. INFECTION CONTROL IN THE WET FINGER ENVIRONMENT (Publishers Press, N. Salt Lake, UT, 1984).

4. *Ibid.*

Chapter Eleven
REVIEW EXERCISES

Date _____ Name_____

Circle the letters of the terms which most closely approximate the answers. There may be one or more than one correct answer. If you circle D, indicate the other answer or answers, if known.

1. Effective instrument recirculation is:

    A. important   B. very important   C. most important

    D. other_____

2. Invasive instruments include:

    A. mouth mirrors   B. carbide burs   C. elevators

    D. other_____

3. Cuts and nicks on personnel's hands occur:

    A. frequently   B. occasionally   C. when they are careless

    D. other_____

4. Once personnel's fingers are cut or nicked, they are:

    A. sore to touch   B. susceptible to infection   C. slow to heal

    D. other_____

5. The most important single goal of instrument recirculation is:

    A. speed   B. efficiency of procedures   C. sterilization of everything
                                                           that can be sterilized

    D. other_____

6. An inviolate rule of instrument recirculation is:

A. never handle con-
taminated instruments
with cut fingers

B. wear latex utility gloves
whenever possible when
handling contaminated
instruments

C. always disinfect counter
tops before placing sterile
instruments down

D. other_____

7. Sterilizer and operator efficiency can be checked by using:

A. sterility assurance
records

B. process indicators

C. biological monitors

D. other_____

8. Covering contaminated instruments in a container with liquid disinfectant will:

A. prevent drying of
blood and serum

B. prevent pathogenic
aerosols

C. make sterilization more
effective

D. other_____

9. Ultrasonic instrument cleaning should be used because:

A. it is faster

B. it is cheaper

C. it is better

D. other_____

10. Instruments should be rinsed after ultrasonic cleaning because rinsing helps to:

A. speed sterilization

B. prevent instrument
spotting in autoclaves

C. prevent residuals on instruments in chemical vapor
sterilizer

D. other_____

11. Sterilized instruments may be stored unpackaged in open drawers only when:

A. no pathogens are
present

B. bags or trays are not handy

C. the doctor says to do so

D. other_____

12. Sterile storage of instruments is possible only in:

    A. bags   B. trays   C. closed drawers

    D. other_____

13. Acceptable methods of storing sterile instruments in trays is in:

    A. closed trays   B. sealed foil   C. see-through trays

    D. other_____

14. The advantage of perforated trays is that they are:

    A. less expensive   B. easily penetrated by steam   C. easier to see inside
                                  and vapors

    D. other_____

15. The advantage of see-through trays is that they are:

    A. less expensive to use   B. easy to stack   C. easier to see inside
       than bags

    D. other_____

16. The biggest disadvantage of bags is that they are:

    A. very expensive   B. limited in size   C. easier to puncture

    D. other_____

17. The advantage of see-through bags is that they are:

    A. easier to seal   B. easier to open   C. opaque

    D. other_____

18. Items too large to fit into bags or trays should be packaged in:

    A. paper wraps   B. hospital-type wraps   C. nylon tubings

    D. other_____

19. Bags should be sealed with:

A. staples   B. tape   C. fast-drying glue

D. other_____

20. Bags will often keep instruments sterile for:

A. weeks   B. months   C. years

D. other_____

21. The sterile storage area should be located:

A. away from busy   B. near instrument recircu-   C. near a disinfectant
   traffic   lation center cleaning area

D. other_____

22. Industrially clean items, if required, should be added to sterile set-up trays:

A. never   B. just before use   C. before storage

D. other_____

23. Bulk packaged items should be handled only with:

A. sterile hands   B. sterile gloves   C. sterile forceps

D. other_____

24. Gauze, cotton rolls and cotton balls should always be:

A. sterile before use   B. pre-packaged   C. disinfected before use

D. other_____

Note: Answers to review exercise are in the back of this book.

Office Design and Choice of Equipment

ABSTRACT: Dentistry is competitive today. Building and equipping a new office or remodeling and re-equipping an existing facility can provide excellent opportunities to raise the health awareness of patients.

Aesthetics, patient appeal and dental productivity should share the spotlight with improved infection control when designing offices and choosing equipment.

Office design is very important in the effectiveness of an infection control program. The ideal is, of course, to begin with new construction that incorporates the latest infection control planning. When this is not practical, established offices can still be re-arranged with certain control goals in mind.

Office Planning and Design

Infection control considerations in the planning, construction, or remodeling of a dental office must anticipate traffic flow, arrangement of treatment and non-treatment areas, choice of materials, and choice of certain types of fixtures and equipment.

Traffic Flow

The treatment areas, laboratory, instrument recirculation center, and other patient handling areas must be effectively separated from the business and patient waiting areas. Patient treatment areas are exposed to the highest number of pathogenic microbes, and every attempt must be made to keep the pathogens where they can be aseptically treated in the quickest, easiest, and most effective ways.

The instrument recirculation center should be separated from the treatment areas and the laboratory. Since all contaminated instruments and materials should be brought to the instrument recirculation center for aseptic treatment and containerized disposal, the instrument recirculation center should not be located where patients are treated. Accordingly, an office plan should incorporate the general design and traffic flow diagrammed in Figure 61.

Choice of Materials

Treatment areas and the laboratory should be designed and constructed to minimize the use of wood surfaces, porous or heavy draperies, and textured wall coverings. Carpet should not be used (see floor coverings on the following pages). Crevices, sharp internal corners, depressions, and other types of construction that potentially collect or protect microbes, should

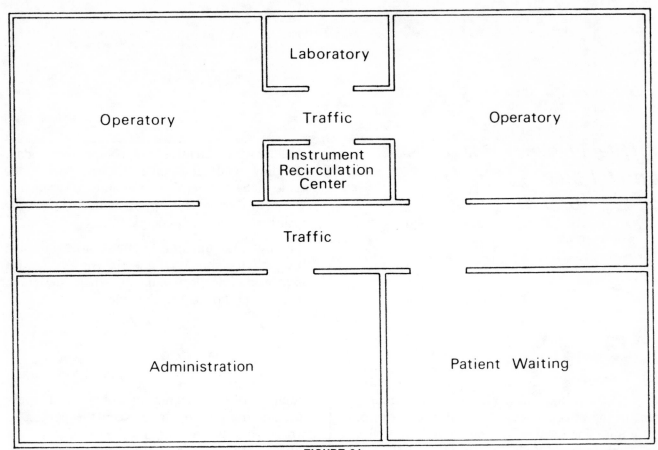

FIGURE 61
Suggested office design and traffic flow.

be avoided. All floors, walls, surfaces, cabinets, drawers, and equipment must be capable of being quickly and easily cleaned and disinfected.

Choice of Fixtures and Equipment

The choice of certain kinds of fixtures and equipment can be very helpful in the control of infection. Following are a few of the important considerations.

Sink Faucets

Sink faucets should be foot, forearm, or electric eye operated. Ideally, hands should never touch faucets, dispensers, or any other part of the body, because the hands offer the greatest probability for re-contamination.

The use of electric eye controlled faucets is becoming more popular. One manufacturer offers a complete line of such controls practical for use in public buildings, hospitals, institutions, and clinics. These faucets are truly "no hands" operations, since water is turned on and off only by movement of the hands near the faucets. See Figure 63.

Dispensers

Soap and lotion dispensers should be foot or forearm actuated and should be wall hung. Portable dispensers placed on work surface tops should be avoided, since they can harbor microbes and interfere with disinfection.

Towel dispensers should be wall hung and of the type which automatically dispense disposable towels without the hands touching a mechanism.

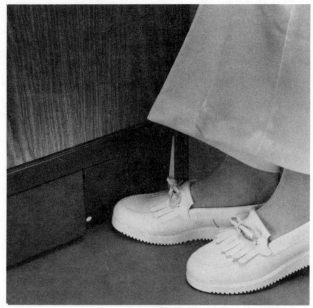

FIGURE 62
Foot control faucet.

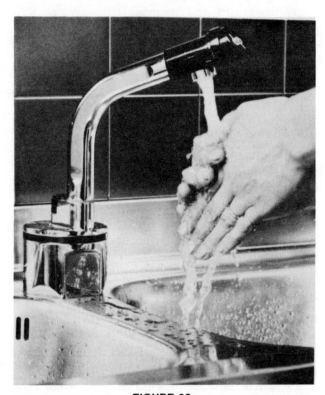

FIGURE 63
Electric eye control faucet requires only movement of hands to activate.

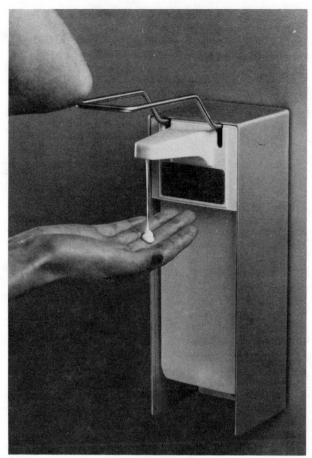

FIGURE 64
''No hands'' soap or lotion dispenser.

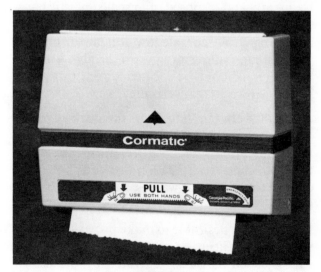

FIGURE 65
''No touch'' towel dispenser.

Waste Containers

The treatment areas, laboratory, and instrument recirculation center should have "hidden" waste receptacles recessed under cabinet tops. Openings should be eight inches or larger in diameter for easy disposal of larger contaminate materials, such as paper towels and 4x4 gauze sponges.

The receptacle should be lined with a disposable plastic bag which can be quickly and easily changed without touching the interior of the bag. A disposable paper bag, such as that used at a hospital bedside, attached to the side of the cabinet by means of adhesive tabs is another alternative. The receptacle in the instrument recirculation center should have a larger capacity than those in the other areas, since much contaminated waste collected in the treatment areas will be brought to the instrument recirculation center for final disposal.

Air Circulation

Air circulation in the office is important to microbial control. Where possible, an office air exchange system should filter all air through microbial filters. The filters should be changed frequently and disposed of in sealed plastic bags. Gloves and a mask should be worn when filters are changed. A separate low volume air evacuation system, pulling air upward through a microbial filter, should be located directly over the instrument recirculation center.

All highly contaminated air should be filtered and vented outside wherever possible so that air from potentially infective treatment areas and the instrument recirculation center is not recirculated to the patient waiting and administration areas.

It is also very desirable to make provision for the venting and filtration of other waste gases and vapors, such as those generated by the use of nitrous oxide and mercury. Strategic placement of filtered vents directly over the areas where amalgam is handled or where nitrous oxide is administered can minimize exposure of staff to potential dangers in the handling of these chemicals.

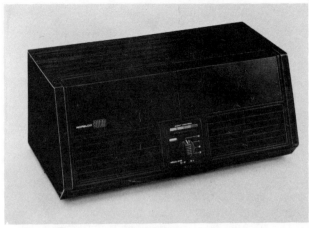

FIGURE 66
Table top office filtration unit.

If an effective central air exchange filtration system is not available, an automatic air sanitizing spray unit or single room air filtration unit should be placed in each room to help reduce microbial count and to mask offensive odors. Air spray units and filtration units contribute to microbial reduction, although they do not disinfect the air.

Floor Coverings

Continuous roll, hard floor covering, such as vinyl, should be used in the treatment areas. Continuous roll eliminates the cracks and crevices of individual square tiles. Floor coverings should be coved to curtail the number of crevices or corners where microbes may accumulate.

While carpet ideally should not be used, there is a strong desire on the part of some practitioners to create with carpeting a "warm" patient atmosphere. When carpet is used, it should not be laid in treatment areas. If laid in other areas, it should be of the low pile synthetic type, sometimes called outdoor or kitchen-type. High pile shag or wool carpet is very difficult to clean and attracts large numbers of microbes.

Choice of Operatory Equipment

In recent years, dental manufacturers have

become more aware of the need to provide equipment which is sterilizable. The most notable example has been the appearance of several models of handpieces which can be sterilized in autoclaves and chemical vapor sterilizers. Use of a wide range of sterilizable equipment will not occur, however, until dentistry makes sterilization a higher priority. Because design and manufacture of new models of products are expensive, industry will not respond until there is sufficient demand from the profession.

In the meantime, when sterilizable equipment is not available, offices must choose equipment which is easily cleaned, disinfected, and/or covered with disposable barriers. Following are some criteria which should be reviewed when purchasing equipment:

1. *Chair*—Should be covered with high quality naugahyde with a minimum of seams. Movements should be controlled by foot. If hand controls are used, they should be of the newer solid state type with a continuous plastic overlay which is easily disinfected.

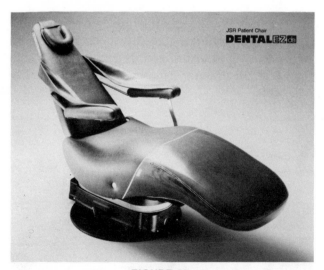

FIGURE 67
Smooth surface chair (preferably without "slings").

2. *Operating Stool*—Should be constructed of same material as chair. If not foot activated, the control lever should be small and easily disinfected or covered with disposable barrier.

3. *Unit*—Should be of smooth construction with a minimum of parts, crevices, cracks, or appendages. Tubings should NOT be mechanically retractable, since mechanical retraction systems protect microbes and are virtually impossible to disinfect. One manufacturer presently offers a non-mechanical retraction system with a tubing retainer which can be removed for disinfection. This method is preferable to mechanical retraction.

Tubings should be straight, not coiled, and should be round on the outside without crevices or depressions.

The unit water supply should be equipped with a vacuum breaker to prevent contaminated water from being pulled back into the syringe or handpieces. This device is present on some units and is available from a few manufacturers. A recent American National Standard/American Dental Association Specification Number 47 includes a paragraph on handpiece coolant water retraction.

The bracket table on the unit should be detachable to allow periodic cleaning and disinfecting.

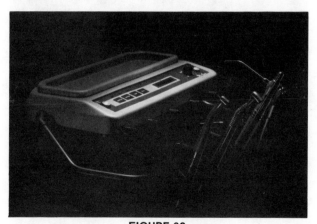

FIGURE 68
Smooth surface unit with disinfectable plastic overlay.

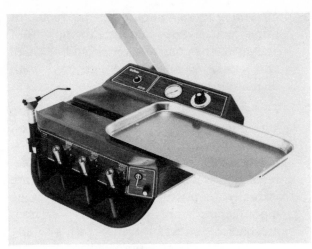

FIGURE 69
Unit with non-mechanical retraction. Tubing retainer is removable for disinfection.

4. *Light*—Should have handles which can be disinfected or covered with a disposable barrier, such as tinfoil. One manufacturer offers presterilized disposable sleeves for use on their fiber optic operating light.

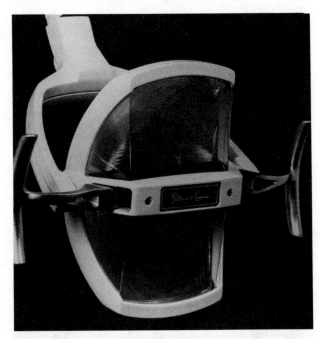

FIGURE 70
Light with handles which can be disinfected or covered.

5. *X-ray*—Controls must be placed outside of the operatory or behind a suitable lead-lined barrier, which allows a safe view of the patient. The overlays for such controls should be of the plastic type for easy disinfection. The actuating switch should be of the hand-held type which can be covered with a disposable barrier.

6. *Handpieces*—Should be fully sterilizable. Easily detached sterilizable tubings are in the development stage and should be used when available.

7. *3-Way Syringe*—Should preferably be fully sterilizable. At least the tip must be easily removable and sterilizable.

8. *Ultrasonic Scaler*—At least the handpiece and tips should be sterilizable.

9. *High Volume Evacuator (HVE), Saliva Ejector, Handpiece, and Other Tubings*—Should be a smooth, non-braided type for easy disinfection. Easily detachable, sterilizable tubings are in the development stage and should be used when available.

10. *Nitrous Oxide Masks*—Should be sterilizable.

    A fully sterilizable nitrous oxide mask and tubings unit has recently been introduced and should be utilized. It is highly desirable that all nitrous "rubber goods" be sterilizable.

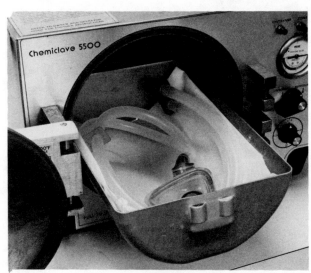

FIGURE 71
Fully sterilizable nitrous system.

162

11. *Emergency Oxygen Masks*—Should be sterilizable. As with nitrous, it is highly desirable that all "rubber goods" be sterilizable because of the high concentrations of body secretions found in the naso-oral region.

The new technology of pressure sensitive switches and microprocessor controlled devices, which have been developed by the computer industry, is in the process of being adapted to some dental equipment. Most of these controls utilize plastic overlays with no cracks, crevices, or protruding parts. Such controls, called membrane switches, are quickly and easily disinfected and are highly desirable for infection control.

Interestingly, equipment which is quickly and most effectively disinfected is often the least expensive because of the simplicity of construction. Also, a wide range of colors, finishes, designs, and configurations are available to assure satisfying aesthetic needs, where appearance is important.

Chapter Twelve
REVIEW EXERCISES

Date _____Name_____

Circle the letters of the terms which most closely approximate the answers. There may be one or more than one correct answer. If you circle D, indicate the other answer or answers, if known.

1. An important goal of dental office design is:

   A. separation of patient treatment areas from non-treatment areas

   B. use of "warm" carpet

   C. use of "warm" wood

   D. other_____

2. The instrument recirculation center should be:

   A. in each treatment area

   B. easily accessible

   C. attractive

   D. other_____

3. Sink faucets should be:

   A. stainless steel

   B. mixer type

   C. "no touch"

   D. other_____

4. Air circulation should be:

   A. filtered

   B. vented outside

   C. fresh

   D. other_____

5. The most desirable floor covering is:

   A. carpet

   B. asphalt tile

   C. continuous vinyl

   D. other_____

6. The most important consideration in the purchase of new dental equipment should be whether it is:

   A. easily disinfected   B. easily cleaned   C. sterilizable when possible

   D. other_____

7. When choosing equipment:

   A. foot activated   B. cloth covered   C. fully disinfectable

   Stools should be:

   A. vinyl covered   B. hydraulic   C. fully disinfectable

   Units should be:

   A. retraction type   B. easily disassembled   C. simple

   Lights should be:

   A. easily disassembled   B. one-piece construction   C. able to be partially covered with a disposable barrier

   X-ray should:

   A. be one-piece construction   B. be sterilizable   C. have portable switch outside operatory area

   Handpieces should be:

   A. sterilizable   B. disinfectable   C. one-piece construction

   3-way syringe should:

   A. be easily disassembled   B. be disinfectable   C. have water retraction

   Ultrasonic scaler should:

   A. be fully sterilizable   B. have removable tip   C. be easily disassembled

Tubings should be:

A. vinyl
B. braided
C. disinfectable

Nitrous oxide masks should be:

A. sterilizable
B. disinfectable
C. made of rubber

8. The best dental equipment for infection control purposes is:

A. simple
B. often less expensive
C. usually more expensive

D. other_____

Note: Answers to review exercises can be found in the back of this book.

CHAPTER 13

Reminders and Summary

ABSTRACT: Improvement requires change. In the case of infection control, the change is a continual process of evolution as new facts and new products are discovered.

Basics should be practiced inviolately, and staff should then build on the basics.

An effective infection control program, in addition to preventing disease, can become a practice-maintaining and practice-building aid.

Dentistry is in a period of infection control transition. Two recent occurrences have catalyzed adoption by most dental treatment staff of at least six basic, routine infection control procedures: (1) wearing gloves; (2) wearing eye protection; (3) wearing masks; (4) sterilizing critical instruments and items; (5) disinfecting touch and splash surfaces; and (6) carefully disposing of contaminated waste. Procedures are being intensified and expanded when treating risk and high risk patients.

The occurrences dramatically changing traditional dentistry's attitude toward the need for infection control were: (1) the Hudson Syndrome—the announcement by Rock Hudson that he had AIDS; and (2) the announcement that a non-high risk dentist had acquired AIDS during routine dental treatment, *without observing basic infection control procedures.*

Dentistry is entering a new era when infection control will become routine and those who do not observe basic procedures will become increasingly visible to concerned patients.

The material in this workbook is intended to teach the basic principles of a comprehensive program of infection control. It is recognized that a significant number of offices may presently practice only a few routine control procedures; therefore, consideration of adoption of even the minimal program may meet with resistance. Comments such as, "Is all this really necessary?" and "It will cost too much" or "I'll have to buy more equipment, supplies, and instruments" and "It's too much trouble" are often heard.

It must be recognized that if dentistry does not promote more effective infection control from within the profession, it will undoubtedly be forced to do so from without by regulatory agencies, governmental agencies, an enlightened lay public, and an aggressive legal system. The recent announcement by OSHA that the basic procedures will be enforced is evidence of government action. Cost must not be a determining factor. Successful defense of one malpractice suit would more than offset the entire cost of an effective infection control program. The circumstances surrounding current infection control are somewhat similar to those of several decades ago when dentistry was suspected of using unsafe x-ray practices resulting in excess radiation to patients. The dental profession, the dental trade, and regulatory agencies worked together to solve the radiation problems, where they existed. The same kind of cooperative effort is needed to solve infection control problems, where they exist.

Dentistry is in a dramatic transition. A number of non-advertising dentists who have practiced in their own solo offices are migrating to practices of multiple dentists in clinics, franchised offices, and advertising groups. The image of dentistry is changing and, at the same time, many established practices are experiencing a reduced patient load. There is opportunity in this changing environment. While effective dental infection control is first a professional, ethical, and moral responsibility, an effective infection control program can also become a valuable aid in the promoting, building, or maintaining of a practice.

Enlightened patients would much rather be treated by concerned health professionals. Patients seek dental care primarily for better health, and such patients are increasingly recognizing the factors that constitute poor, average, or good treatment. Inadequate infection control is becoming increasingly visible, and effective infection control is becoming increasingly appreciated. The sooner a more effective control program is started, the sooner the practice-building bonus can be realized.

At the same time that it is highly desirable, if not mandatory, to adopt and then improve infection control procedures, it is also advisable not to attempt too much too quickly. Personnel need to master an orderly step-by-step program. Such personnel may become discouraged if pushed too quickly. Parts of the minimal program should be practiced first, and then new procedures should be added until they become routine. Once minimal procedures are learned, advancement to a routine program is relatively easy.

This workbook is designed to instruct the reader in the basics of an effective infection control program. The information, however, is intended to serve only as a foundation for further building and strengthening of the program through additions contributed by the inventiveness of dentists and their staffs. Improvements in the program are to be encouraged, but the basics must be retained to serve as the continuing foundation for the evolving program.

The tables on the following pages summarize certain of the information previously presented in the basic program. Such tables should be posted as reminders to all staff.

Summary

In a perfect world, it would be ideal to eliminate all pathogenic microbes from the dental environment, but such a goal is not attainable. Fortunately, it is also unnecessary to reach this level of perfection. An infection control program is considered effective when the number of microbes remaining in the office is reduced to as low a level as possible. When this is accomplished, pathogens introduced to patients or personnel may be overcome through function of the normal body defenses.

A program takes months, even years, to refine to full effectiveness. Personnel should be trained to learn a new procedure as soon as a previous one has been mastered. Success is fulfilling and will encourage staff to develop new techniques, new approaches, and constantly better control. The process should be unending. New discoveries offer advancements in the state-of-the-art. Change is mandatory because infection control is an evolving, changing skill.

Infection control should be viewed as a challenging occupation in which the rewards are great — sometimes even life-saving.

TABLE 15
SOME INFECTION CONTROL REMINDERS

DO	DON'T
1. Do clean and disinfect floors, cabinets, sinks, etc., as required, with an effective surface disinfectant.	1. Don't delegate duties to janitorial services without providing supervision.
2. Do use heavy utility gloves when handling contaminated instruments.	2. Don't let blood dry on instruments.
3. Do clean and disinfect work surfaces, bracket tables, chair arms, light handles, etc., between patients.	3. Don't use 2x2 gauze sponge technique.
4. Do cover headrest, bracket table, light handles, x-ray head, etc. with disposables.	4. Don't re-use covers.
5. Do flush water in unit and other equipment for ten minutes before first use.	5. Don't invite stagnation.
6. Do disinfect HVE system daily.	6. Don't invite stagnation.
7. Do wear masks for all procedures.	7. Don't use just any mask.
8. Do wear protective glasses.	8. Don't rub eyes.
9. Do use gloves, especially on emergency and high risk patients.	9. Don't re-use non-sterile gloves.
10. Do multiple wash-rinse of hands between patients.	10. Don't touch faucet handles, re-use towels, or re-use soap.
11. Do have patient multiple rinse mouth before treatment.	11. Don't do intensive dentistry on patients who have not rinsed.
12. Do use disposables whenever possible.	12. Don't re-use disinfected disposables.
13. Do ultrasonically clean instruments whenever possible.	13. Don't hand scrub instruments, especially without heavy gloves.
14. Do sterilize all non-disposable instruments and items possible.	14. Don't use cold disinfectants for instruments which can be heat sterilized.
15. Do disinfect only those items which cannot be sterilized.	15. Don't use disinfectants too long without changing.

TABLE 15 (Continued)

DO	DON'T
16. Do use only EPA/ADA disinfectants.	16. Don't use "quats" or alcohol.
17. Do "package" instruments for storage.	17. Don't use a "package" which interferes with sterilization.
18. Do choose effective sterilizer(s).	18. Don't compromise on the purchase of sterilizer(s) because of cost.
19. Do maintain sterilizers.	19. Don't allow inexperienced servicing.
20. Do use a process indicator with each sterilization load.	20. Don't be confused by a "specialized" indicator.
21. Do use a biological monitor at least monthly.	
22. Do maintain a sterility assurance file.	
23. Do purchase equipment which is sterilizable or easily disinfectable.	23. Don't sacrifice cleanability for aesthetics.
24. Do train personnel to think "cross-contamination."	24. Don't delegate to untrained personnel.
25. Do train personnel to think "sterilization."	25. Don't delegate to untrained personnel.
26. Do train personnel to think "legality."	26. Don't delegate to untrained personnel.

TABLE 16
STERILIZATION DISINFECTION GUIDE

Items	Autoclave	Chemical Vapor Sterilizer	Dry Heat Sterilizer	Glutaralde-hydes	Disinfectants	Disposables
Air-water Syringe	2	1			3	
Air-water Tip	1	1				
Bite Blocks	1	1				
Burs		1				
Cloth Packs	1					
Cotton & Gauze—Small Amounts	1	2				
Cotton & Gauze—Large Amounts	1					
Counter Tops					1	
Endodontic Kits		1	2			
Handpieces—Sterilizable	2	1				
Handpieces—Non-sterilizable				1	3	
HVE Tips						1
Impression Trays—Metal	1	1				
Instruments—Carbon Steel		1				
Instruments—Stainless Steel	2	1	3			
Instruments—Surgical	2	1	3			
Light Handles					3	1
Matrix Bands						1
Matrix Retainers	2	1	3			
Needles, Anesthetic						1
Needles, Suture		1				
Periodontal Curettes		1				
Prophy Cups				3		1
Prophy Angles	2	1				
Prostheses, Metallic				1	3	
Prostheses, Non-metallic				1	3	
Rag Wheels	1					
Reamers and Files		1	2			
Rubber Dam Clamps, Forceps and Frames	2	1				
Rubber Dam						1
Saliva Ejectors						1
Sharpening Stones	1	1				
Syringes—Plastic						1
Syringes—Metal	2	1				
X-ray Film Positioners					1	3
X-ray Switch					3	1

Legend: 1—Best   2—Good   3—Acceptable   Blank—Not Recommended

Chapter Three:
1-C; 2-A; 3-C; 4-B; 5-A; 6-C, D (sterile); 7-B; 8-C; 9-B; 10-B; 11-C; 12-B; 13-A, B, C,D; 14-C; 15-A; 16-A, B, C, D; 17-C; 18-B, C; 19-B; 20-D (contamination from one person to another).

Chapter Four:
1-A, C; 2-B, C, D (many); 3-D (easier to identify); 4-A, D (harder to identify); 5-C; 6-C; 7-A; 8-C; 9-C; 10-A; 11-A, B,C, D (all potential infections); 12-A, C, D (personnel infection); 13-A, C; 14-A, B, C, D (others).

Chapter Five:
1-B, D (mature, etc.); 2-B, D (microbiology, etc.); 3-C; 4-C; 5-A; 6-B; 7-B; 8-A; 9-A, B, C; 10-B, C; 11-A; 12-B; 13-A, B; 14-A, B, C, D (many precautions); 15-C; 16-A; 17-A, B; 18-D (only once when absolutely necessary); 19-C; 20-B; 21-A, A, C, C, B, A, C, D (disinfect eyeglasses), B, C.

Chapter Six:
1-A, C; 2-B; 3-A; 4-A, B, C; 5-A, B, C; 6-A; 7-B; 8-A, B, C; 9-D (sterilized daily); 10-A, B; 11-A, C; 12-C.

Chapter Seven:
1-B; 2-A, B; 3-B, C; 4-B; 5-C; 6-C; 7-C; 8-C; 9-A; 10-A; 11-A, C; 12-B; 13-A, B, C; 14-A, D (many items); 15-B; 16-C; 17-A, C; 18-B, D (commercial needle destroyer).

Chapter Eight:
1-A, B; 2-C; 3-B; 4-D (FDA); 5-C; 6-A; 7-C.

Chapter Nine:
1-C; 2-D (glutaraldehyde); 3-A; 4-C, D (Items which cannot be sterilized. In place of disposable or barrier.); 5-C, D (all chemical sterilants and disinfectants); 6-A, B, C; 7-A, B, C; 8-A, B; 9-B; 10-A, D (15-40 minutes); 11-B, D (2 hours); 12-A, B; 13-A, C; 14-B; 15-B, C; 16-A; 17-B; 18-B, C; 19-A, B; 20-C; 21-B; 22-B; 23-A; 24-B, C; 25-C; 26-B; 27-B; 28-C; 29-B; 30-A, B; 31-B; 32-A, C; 33-B; 34-A, B; 35-B; 36-A; 37-A; 38-A; 39-C; 40-B; 41-A; 42-C; 43-C; 44-A; 45-D (none); 46-B; 47-C.

Chapter Ten:
1-A; 2-C; 3-A, B, C; 4-B, C, D (foot operated); 5-C; 6-C.

Chapter Eleven:
1-C; 2-B, C, D (many); 3-A; 4-B; 5-C; 6-B; 7-C; 8-A, C; 9-A, C; 10-B, C; 11-C; 12-A, B, D (wraps); 13-A, C; 14-B; 15-A, C; 16-B, C; 17-D (easy to see into); 18-A; 19-B, D (self-sealing); 20-A, B; 21-A; 22-B; 23-B, C; 24-A.

Chapter Twelve:
1-A; 2-D (separated from treatment areas); 3-C; 4-A, B, C (sometimes); 5-C; 6-A, B; 7-A, A, C, C, C, A, B, C, A; 8-A, B.

NOTES

NOTES

NOTES

NOTES

NOTES

NOTES